Stroke Services

Policy and practice across Europe

Edited by
Charles Wolfe
Christopher McKevitt
and
Anthony Rudd

Radcli... ...ess

Radcliffe Medical Press Ltd
18 Marcham Road
Abingdon
Oxon OX14 1AA
United Kingdom

www.radcliffe-oxford.com
The Radcliffe Medical Press electronic catalogue and online ordering facility.
Direct sales to anywhere in the world.

British Library Cataloguing in Publication Data

A catalogue record for this book is available from the British Library.

ISBN 1 85775 455 7

Typeset by Aarontype Ltd, Easton, Bristol
Printed and bound by TJ International Ltd, Padstow, Cornwall

Contents

See www.radcliffe-oxford.com/stroke for the appendices containing the forms required to build a workable data set.

List of contributors

Roger Beech
Department of Operational Research, University of Keele, Keele, UK

Ajay Bhalla
Department of Public Health Sciences, Guy's, King's and St Thomas' School of Medicine, London, UK

Anna Czlonkowska
Institute of Psychiatry and Neurology, Warsaw, Poland

Ruth Dundas
Department of Public Health Sciences, Guy's, King's and St Thomas' School of Medicine, London, UK

Shah Ebrahim
Department of Social Medicine, University of Bristol, Bristol, UK

Maurice Giroud
Servie de Neurologie, Hopital General, Dijon, France

Richard Grieve
Department of Public Health Sciences, Guy's, King's and St Thomas' School of Medicine, London, UK

Gerald Haidinger
Institute of Tumor Biology and Cancer Research, Vienna, Austria

Peter Heuschmann
Department of Neurology and Public Health, University of Erlangen-Nuremberg, Germany

Walter Holland
Emeritus Professor of Public Health Medicine, UMDS, St Thomas' Hospital, London, UK

Domenico Inzitari
Dipartimento di Scienze Neurologiche e Psichiatriche, Ospedale Careggi, Florence, Italy

Peter Kolominsky
Department of Neurology and Public Health, University of Erlangen-Nuremberg, Germany

Klaus Kunze
Department of Neurology, University of Hamburg, Hamburg, Germany

Christopher McKevitt
Department of Public Health Sciences, Guy's, King's and St Thomas' School of Medicine, London, UK

Mehool Patel
Department of Public Health Sciences, Guy's, King's and St Thomas' School of Medicine, London, UK

Ilona Purina
Latvian Neuroangiological Centre, Riga Seventh Clinical Hospital, Riga, Latvia

Daiva Rastenyte
Institute of Cardiology, Kaunas Medical Academy, Kaunas Lithuania

India Remedios
Department of Rehabilitation Medicine, Hospital Garcia, Almada, Portugal

Anthony Rudd
Department of Care of the Elderly, Guy's and St Thomas' Hospitals Trust, London, UK

Danuta Ryglewicz
Institute of Psychiatry and Neurology, Warsaw, Poland

Kate Tilling
Department of Public Health Sciences, Guy's, King's and St Thomas' School of Medicine, London, UK

Matias Torrent
Health Care Research Unit, Menorca, Spain

Charles Wolfe
Department of Public Health Sciences, Guy's, King's and St Thomas' School of Medicine, London, UK

Introduction

There are significant disparities in health outcomes and access to healthcare in Europe. For example, the health of Central and Eastern Europe continues to lag well behind that in the West. There is also a distinct North–South pattern of inequalities within Europe. There is a lack of policies for identifying the threats to health, and often an absence of interventions required to overcome these obstacles.

Survival rates for major diseases such as cancer and stroke vary dramatically between countries. What drives such inequalities cannot be simply explained. Factors such as wealth and socio-economic status have a bearing on life expectancy, but there are also other significant influences on health outcome. Across Europe there will be a range of patterns of healthcare services for different diseases. Some of these differences in provision will be appropriate, reflecting differences in the health economy of the country, whereas others may be inappropriate.

To inform policy makers, much needs to be understood about the relationship between a country and its culture, specific diseases and healthcare interventions. In this book we illustrate how groups of clinicians and health service researchers have started to address these issues for stroke. Stroke is a disease that is a major health challenge for Europe – it is the third commonest cause of death, and is a disease which will become more common with an ageing population. There are many factors that impinge on the outcomes for stroke patients, one of which is the level of healthcare provided. The different aspects of stroke care include primary prevention, acute management, rehabilitation, secondary prevention and longer-term care.

Clinicians who are interested in assessing the quality of their services, as well as health service researchers and policy makers require at least some of the tools used in health service research, but they may not have them to hand or know where to find them. This book will:

- demonstrate methodologies and selected findings of a European study designed to evaluate stroke
- use stroke as a case study to reflect the breadth of issues relevant to health services research. In this context we take health services research to include describing and comparing structures, processes and outcomes of healthcare.

• focus in particular on issues of comparison of process and outcome between centres and countries.

The book has been written by members of European Union Biomed-funded research projects and edited by the co-ordinating centre. The book aims to address the following issues:

• how to interpret variations in health status
• how to build a workable data set to answer questions (*see* www.radcliffe-oxford.com/stroke)
• how to set up a population disease register
• how to measure the quality of service provision (structure and process)
• how to interpret outcome
• how to incorporate subjective outcome assessment into evaluations
• how to cost care across countries
• how to identify the benefits and hurdles to multicentre European research.

It is hoped that the reader will find this book useful not only for stroke research but also to enable them to use the generic tools and principles described and apply them to other diseases. This book provides a practical example of what can be achieved in European research, and as such it is not a textbook. It identifies the benefits and disadvantages of European research and is pragmatic in its approach to addressing health services research issues. The results of the European stroke collaboration pose as many questions as they set out to answer, but the book highlights the value of researchers and clinicians from many countries joining together to address important questions that could not be answered at a national level.

Charles Wolfe
August 2001

Overview: measuring quality of healthcare

Walter W Holland CBE FFPHM FRCP

This book tackles two 'holy grails' namely the measurement of quality of healthcare and international comparisons of healthcare. It uses the variations in healthcare for stroke illness in a number of European countries to suggest possibilities and methods for linking the processes of care to the outcomes of healthcare.

International comparisons in epidemiology have a long tradition. The International Epidemiological Association, which has as one of its objectives the fostering of research internationally to improve both knowledge and practice, at its Fourth International Scientific Conference in Princeton, New Jersey, in 1964 considered this topic in some depth, and selected papers were published.[1]

The Princeton meeting considered many of the issues raised in this book. Two underlying themes emerged. First, since many conditions and their causes transcend national boundaries, control efforts must be made on the basis of common definitions or techniques. Secondly, many conditions show distinct differences in rates of incidence, cerebral haemorrhage being one example which was given, but methods need to be developed to ensure that these differences are real and not artefacts of the method of measurement.

Comparisons of conditions both within and between countries imply that uniform terms are used, so that one is comparing like with like. Part of this process concerns the definition of words and concepts before studies are undertaken in different locations or cultures. Although this methodology has been used in this investigation, it is important to appreciate that complete agreement is never likely. This has been shown in many studies, ranging from investigations of diarrhoea[2] to chronic respiratory disease.[3] Similarly, the use of diagnoses in cross-national comparisons is just as susceptible to variability.[4] To complement these types of measurement, the use of 'hard' data (e.g. electrocardiogram, blood pressure, X-ray) has been suggested and employed by workers such as Cochrane[5] and Higgins.[6] The advantage of these is that the recordings can be interpreted in more than one place, so that there is greater assurance about the comparability of findings from one place to another. However, even with all of these caveats, there are many international studies which have shown that carefully recorded information on disease in different countries is reasonably reliable in highlighting differences in frequency, care processes and outcome between countries.

There have been several international comparisons of health services or disease processes. The latter are relatively easy to execute so long as comparable populations and methods of measurement are used. Examples include the studies by Keys and his colleagues[7] of cardiovascular disease in the USA and several European countries, by Comstock et al.[8] and Holland and Reid[9,10] of chronic respiratory and cardiovascular disease in the UK, USA and Japan, and by Burney[11] of asthma in Europe. An example of the comparison of outcomes of health services in Europe is provided by the studies of avoidable mortality co-ordinated by Holland.[12] International comparison of the provision of health services for specific conditions is best illustrated by the work of Kohn and White.[13] However, this is probably the first study comparing both the process of healthcare and the outcome in several European countries. It thus attempts to identify the components of health service quality.

Healthcare quality depends on a variety of factors, the most important of which are as follows:

- access to care — this depends both on the availability of services and on their utilisation
- the speed and process of response to the problem — in an acute condition such as stroke, patients, family members, neighbours and health service providers need to recognise the occurrence of a problem and respond appropriately to it
- the appropriateness of the process of response (e.g. speed of admission to hospital and stroke unit, administration of appropriate drugs, relevant laboratory and imaging investigation, etc.)
- the appropriateness of both immediate and long-term treatment, including rehabilitation (e.g. on a stroke unit)
- the outcome of the treatment (e.g. death, recovery, disability, etc.) and, of course, the satisfaction of the patient with the treatment given.

This study provides information on all of these aspects, and the authors discuss the implications of their findings. In view of the differences they have found both in the processes of care and in the outcome of comparable patients in different locations, important questions arise as to what can and will be done to improve the services for stroke. Although it is very likely that these studies do provide an accurate picture of the situation in various parts of Europe, none the less it is necessary to proceed with caution when advising on alterations in health service provision. There are two further crucial questions which need to be answered.

The first relates to the representativeness of the findings in the institutions surveyed, compared with other institutions in the same country. The second question is even more difficult. The study was based on secondary care institutions, and epidemiologists are aware of the problem of extrapolating findings from investigations on selected cases rather than defined populations. Thus the importance for health policy of the findings of major differences in the outcome of care both between and within countries would be greatly enhanced if further research was conducted on the outcome of stroke illnesses in several defined populations in each country.

The methodology described and the results obtained provide an excellent example of how international comparative studies can assist in the improvement of outcome for an important disease, but as with all such studies, further questions are raised and these need to be answered.

References

1 Acheson RM (ed.) (1965) *Comparability in International Epidemiology.* Millbank Memorial Fund, New York.

2 Cvjetanovic B, Kaufman P and van Ziyk WJ (1965) Diarrhoeal diseases, international cross-sectional studies. In: RM Acheson (ed.) *Comparability in International Epidemiology.* Millbank Memorial Fund, New York, 240–54.

3 Holland WW (1965) Chronic respiratory diseases – the rationale of field surveys. In: RM Acheson (ed.) *Comparability in International Epidemiology.* Millbank Memorial Fund, New York, 77–89.

4 Kelson MC and Heller RF (1983) The effect of death certification and coding practices on observed differences in respiratory disease mortality in eight EEC countries. *Rev Epidemiol Sante Publ.* **31**: 423–32.

5 Cochrane AL (1965) Studies of a total community – Rhondda Fach, S Wales. In: RM Acheson (ed.) *Comparability in International Epidemiology.* Millbank Memorial Fund, New York, 326–32.

6 Higgins ITT (1965) Ischaemic heart disease. In: RM Acheson (ed.) *Comparability in International Epidemiology.* Millbank Memorial Fund, New York, 23–31.

7 Keys A and White PD (eds) (1956) *World Trends in Cardiology. I. Cardiovascular epidemiology.* Paul B Hoeber, New York.

8 Comstock GW, Stone RW, Sakai Y, Matsuya T and Tonascia JA (1973) Respiratory findings and urban living. *Arch Environ Health.* **27**: 143–50.

9   Holland WW, Reid DD, Seltser R and Stone RW (1965) Respiratory disease in England and the United States. *Arch Environ Health*. **10**: 338–43.

10   Reid DD, Holland WW and Rose GA (1967) An Anglo-American cardiovascular comparison. *Lancet*. **2**: 1375–8.

11   Burney P (1998) Ten years of research on asthma in Europe. The European Community Health Survey. *Rev Epidemiol Sante Publ*. **46**: 491–6.

12   Holland WW (ed.) (1988, 1991, 1993 and 1997) *The European Community Atlas of 'Avoidable Death'* (1e); Volume I (2e); Volume II (2e, 3e). Oxford University Press, Oxford.

13   Kohn R and White KL (1976) *Health Care: an international study*. Oxford University Press, Oxford.

CHAPTER 1

The problem of interpreting variations in health status (morbidity and mortality) in Europe

Maurice Giroud, Anna Czlonkowska, Danuta Ryglewicz and Charles Wolfe

Variations in morbidity and mortality: problems of interpretation

The chances of dying from a given disease vary enormously from one country to another.[1,2] Such variations in death rates are to a large extent unexplained, but they may be due to differences in the following:

- the health status of the population
- the prevalence of risk factors for the disease and hence the incidence of the disease
- access to care and ways of managing the disease
- the way in which death is coded and recorded.

The measurement of health outcomes of populations or individuals is fundamental to understanding their needs, planning health services and possibly thereby reducing mortality. However, it is important to remember that many factors other than medical care may influence health status. Such factors include sociodemography (e.g. age, gender, social class influencing access to resources), environment, case severity, comorbidity and clinical management.

This book focuses on stroke, but it also treats stroke as a model for studying the variation in outcome between countries and the consequences of chronic diseases in general. Stroke provides a good example of a chronic disease of social and economic significance for a number of reasons. It is the third commonest cause of death worldwide, responsible for around 5.5 million deaths a year. In the developed world stroke ranks third after myocardial infarction and cancer, accounting for around 10–12% of deaths. It is estimated that around 1 million ischaemic strokes occur in Europe each year,[1,2] and nearly 400 000 patients die in Europe each year as a consequence of stroke.[2] Stroke is also one of the commonest causes of adult physical disability. The management of stroke and its consequences consumes a considerable amount of health service resources. For example, it has been estimated that stroke care accounts for almost 6% of National Health and Social Service expenditure in the UK.[3]

Mortality data are the most readily available figures on health status in many countries, and are therefore used as indicators of the state of health of a population. However, for a disease such as stroke, which is responsible for significant long-term disability, it is important that other outcome domains, such as impairment, disability and handicap, are also measured.

The extent of variation in outcome of stroke

Are death rates declining? There are important issues to consider when comparing disease-specific mortality rates across regions and countries. There will be differences in the age–sex structure of the populations that may account for some or all of the observed differences. Although the reduction of overall death rates for a disease is important, the focus needs to be on reducing premature mortality and morbidity. In most industrialised countries, stroke mortality declined for several decades. In the USA the decline in age-adjusted stroke mortality began in 1918. Despite a general decline in mortality from stroke in Western Europe, there is considerable variation in the rate of decline between countries, and in Eastern Europe mortality rates are either stable or increasing.[4] Data comparing death rates in the 1980s with those in the early 1990s in populations aged under 75 years show that in those countries with low mortality rates the decreases were most marked. Countries such as Japan, Australia and France had reductions of around 5–8% per year. In other Western European countries, the rate of decline has been 2–4% annually, with the decline affecting men and women in all age groups. In contrast, those former Eastern European countries with high mortality rates showed increases of around 2–4% per year over the same time period[4] (see Figure 1.1).

Recently published statistics suggest that the long-term decline in stroke mortality rates may have ceased. Wolfe and Burney[5] indicated in an age-period cohort analysis of stroke mortality in England and Wales that mortality rates may be increasing in younger cohorts, which will have an effect on overall death rates in the next few decades. In the USA,

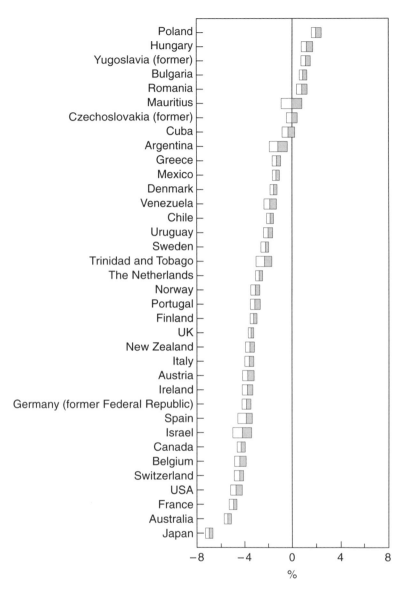

Figure 1.1   Annual percentage change in mortality from stroke in men aged 35–74 years in selected countries during the entire study period of 1968–94. (*Source*: Sarti C *et al.*[4] Reproduced with permission.)

age-adjusted stroke mortality rates increased between 1992 and 1993, and a recent report documented another rise in the preliminary rate for 1995. Age-adjusted rates per 100 000 population for the years 1991 to 1995 were 26.8, 26.2, 26.5, 26.5 and 26.7, respectively.[6] In addition, the demographic change associated with a rapidly ageing population in Europe, which is already creating a crisis in both the healthcare and social care sectors, means

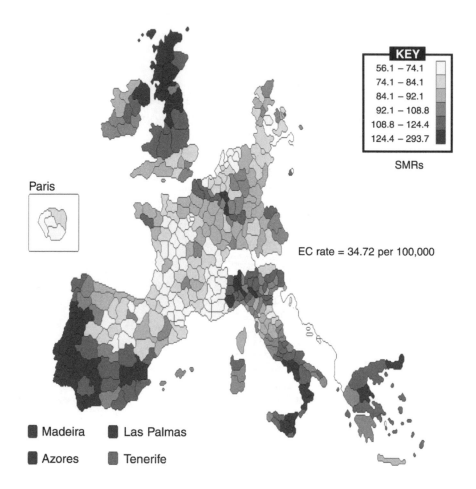

Figure 1.2 Hypertensive and cerebrovascular disease mortality for individuals aged 35–64 years during the period 1985–89. (*Source*: Holland WW.[7] Reproduced with permission.)

that despite a stable or downward trend in mortality, numbers in real terms are likely to increase over the next few decades.

What is the extent of the variation in mortality? A previous European Union Biomed Programme published atlases of 'avoidable deaths' in the European population aged under 65 years, including deaths resulting from hypertensive disease and stroke.[7] Figure 1.2 shows the significant variation in standardised mortality ratios for hypertension and stroke.

Data provided by the World Health Organisation demonstrate an eight-fold variation in stroke mortality rates between countries among both men and women.[1,2] In Europe, the age-adjusted stroke mortality rate ranges from 30 to 250 per 100 000 population, and in the USA it ranges from 50 to 100 per 100 000.[8] Stroke mortality rates calculated on the basis of stroke events registered in the MONICA Project, together with age-standardised mortality rates derived from official statistics (ICD codes 430–438), show that stroke mortality was higher in Yugoslavia, Poland, Lithuania, Finland and the Russian Federation than in Italy, Germany, Denmark and Sweden.[9-11] In all cases rates are 25–50% higher for men than for women, and countries with high rates for men also have high rates among women.[9-11]

These variations in the rate of decline in stroke mortality and in overall stroke mortality rates raise many questions (*see* Box 1.1). For a chronic disease such as stroke, mortality is not the only outcome measure that needs to be addressed. We need to know what drives these differences in mortality, be they related to factors associated with the risk of having a stroke in the first place or factors that influence survival after the stroke.

Box 1.1   The current unanswered questions

- What are the variations in mortality and morbidity from stroke in Europe?
- What influences these variations?
- How can these questions be addressed in an international context?

The next few pages outline what is known about some of the factors that influence stroke mortality.

Variations in incidence

Although mortality data are commonly used to describe the risk of stroke in a population, incidence is a more sensitive indicator. This is because incidence is influenced by the prevalence of risk factors in the population, whereas mortality rates are also influenced by differences in stroke severity and by healthcare.

Stroke incidence measures

One advantage of measuring the incidence of stroke is the potential of community-based studies to answer additional questions based on an unbiased sample of incidence cases.[12] These may include follow-up for outcome in terms of case fatality, recurrence and disability, case–control studies of various risk factors, and assessment of stroke services (*see* Chapter 3).

A careful choice of study design is crucial to ensure that the identified aims are achieved without the collection of excess useless data which simply create extra work for the investigators and may compromise the quality of the study.

There have been a number of comparative studies of incidence rates both internationally and in Europe specifically, but methodological differences make comparisons across studies difficult. For example, studies have focused on particular age groups, have compared different time periods and used different means of ascertaining and diagnosing stroke. Therefore some of the reported variations have biases resulting from the methodologies employed.[9,12] Generally, however, there is little dramatic variation in the overall incidence of stroke in Europe. This is perhaps not surprising, since all of the populations studied were predominantly white with a westernised lifestyle. A persistent finding of the Dijon incidence studies in France has been strikingly low rates. This could be an artefact due to methodological differences, most probably in case finding, but it raises the possibility of the so-called 'French paradox', namely low rates of cardiovascular disease and stroke in France, attributed by some to wine consumption.[13-15] Further reliable stroke incidence studies from this part of the world are needed to investigate this possibility further, as Dijon may be unrepresentative of France in general. At the other extreme, the high incidence rates in Novosibirsk in Russia may also be due to methodological artefact, or they may indicate a real difference reflecting a higher level of population risk factors for stroke. However, stroke rates in Novosibirsk do not rank as high in the elderly, and the reasons for this are not clear. Perhaps case finding among older people in this population was less efficient. Another possibility is that there are fewer stroke-prone individuals in this age group because of earlier deaths from complications of ischaemic heart disease in a population with a high prevalence of risk factors for both cardiovascular and cerebrovascular disease. As a rule, individual regions may be unrepresentative of their country, and before comparing disease-specific mortality rates, it would be wise to compare total mortality rates and proportional mortality rates between regions. In this way disease-specific rates can be interpreted within a wider context.

A report of the WHO MONICA Project stated that age-standardised stroke incidence rates per 100 000 population aged 35–64 years ranged from 137 to 388 in men and from 69 to 175 in women, which may in part explain the variations in mortality in this age group.[11] The approximately 2.5-fold difference between stroke incidence in Dijon, France and Novosibirsk, Russia is considerably less than the approximately eight-fold difference in mortality (from official statistics) between France and Russia.[1] Although it is possible that the much larger mortality difference could be due to a higher case fatality rate in Russia, another potential explanation is that mortality statistics are simply not reliable enough to reflect international variation in stroke incidence accurately. The question raised is whether mortality rates are driven by the incidence of the disease or case fatality.

With regard to pathological subtypes of stroke, no striking differences in distribution have been observed between populations, but the studies contributing to the analysis are again drawn from broadly similar types of population. Studies from the Far East show a similar overall incidence rate of stroke to other parts of the world. These include the WHO MONICA project,[16] a study from Beijing, China[17] and the review of Malmgren and colleagues in 1987,[18] which included an incidence study from Shibata, Japan conducted in the 1970s.[19] However, most of the Far Eastern studies have suggested that the proportion of intracerebral haemorrhages is significantly higher (by up to 35%) than in white populations.[20] Unfortunately, none of these investigations fulfils our criteria for an ideal study, and therefore we cannot confirm that this excess of haemorrhages is real. This would require studies employing comparable methods and with high rates of accurate pathological diagnosis. Therefore a further point to consider when interpreting mortality rates is the type of stroke and its severity.

There have been no long-term incidence studies with enough power to explain the fall in mortality in the last 40 years. In general, since the late 1950s incidence rates for stroke have been declining, at least in Japan, the USA and some Western European countries, although in the last few years the end of this long-term decline in stroke incidence has been observed. The most frequently quoted data come from Rochester in the USA.[21] In the Rochester study, the incidence of first-ever stroke decreased until the end of the 1970s in all age and sex groups. The rate fell from 205 per 100 000 in the period 1955–59 to 128 per 100 000 in the period 1975–79. However, for the period 1985–89, although the incidence of untreated hypertension was stable or even decreasing, the incidence rate of stroke was 13% higher (153 per 100 000) than in 1975–79. This rate remained relatively constant (145 per 100 000) from 1985 to 1989.[21] Similar findings were reported from Frederiksberg in Denmark for men aged 65–84 years, when comparing the two periods 1972–74 and 1989–90.[22] The WHO MONICA data also suggested a decline in stroke incidence rates among men in 13 populations and among women in 15 of the 17 MONICA populations. Other studies reported slight increases in incidence, although some countries with high incidence rates, such as Russia and Finland, reported a decline over the period 1982–92.[23–25]

During the last two decades the changes in stroke incidence have not been identical in men and women. In Auckland in New Zealand, incidence rates increased among women aged under 75 years and deceased in men aged over 75 years.[24] In Denmark, between 1976 and 1993 the stroke incidence remained stable among men aged 45–64 years and women aged 45–84 years, whereas a significant decrease was found in men aged 65–84 years.[25] In Sweden, data from the Northern Sweden MONICA stroke register suggested that stroke incidence decreased in men aged under 65 years, increased in those aged 65–74 years, and remained unchanged in women.[26] However, in some other Swedish studies, trends of increasing incidence rates among women have been reported.[27] These observations cannot easily be explained. Analysis of data from community-based studies in Eastern Finland suggests that the decrease in the prevalence of hypertension and smoking between 1972 and 1977 accounts for about 30% of the decline in stroke events.[28] It has been suggested that improved treatment of hypertension, improved metabolic control of diabetes and the use of antithrombotic therapy in patients at high risk of embolic stroke has led to a reduction in the incidence of stroke.[29] At the same time, better treatment of cardiac diseases has increased the number of people at high risk of stroke.[6] Changes in particular behaviours, especially among women in European countries, may also be responsible for the increased stroke incidence.[27] For example, in recent years the proportion of Danish men aged 65 years or older who smoke has been stable or decreased, whereas the proportion of Danish women aged 65 years or older who smoke has increased.[25]

Future collaborative comparisons should ideally address incidence and case fatality from stroke in prospective studies using similar methodologies. This may eventually help us to determine whether international mortality differences are due to differences in incidence, case fatality, or both, or whether they are just an artefact. Only in this way will it be possible to improve our knowledge of the aetiology and prevention of the third commonest cause of death in the Western world. Chapter 3 outlines the principles involved in establishing such studies.

Specific studies investigating the reasons for variations in morbidity and mortality rates

In developed countries there are significant variations in the age- and sex-standardised stroke death rates both between and within countries. Figure 1.2 illustrates the standardised mortality ratio differences in younger people (under 65 years of age) in a previous European Union-funded Biomed programme.

The usefulness of monitoring time trends in mortality rates, particularly avoidable deaths in younger people (under 65 years) has been addressed. Mackenbach and colleagues[30] reviewed many studies that have attempted to explain variations in mortality between countries. They concluded that time trends showed that avoidable mortality had declined faster in recent decades than most other causes of death. Studies of geographical variation have shown that avoidable mortality is consistently associated with socio-economic factors, and that the association with the provision of healthcare resources was weak and inconsistent. Mackenbach and colleagues also suggested that in-depth studies at an individual level were more likely to produce information about factors that limit the effectiveness of health services than further studies of aggregate data.

The decline in stroke mortality observed in many countries reflects an improvement in stroke case fatality rates rather than a decline in the incidence of stroke. In most countries, stroke case fatality rates have decreased over the last 40–50 years. In Rochester there was a reduction in 30-day case fatality following stroke (all types combined) from 33% in 1945–49 to 17% in 1980–84, with marked differences within stroke subgroups, particularly for cerebral haemorrhage.[8] In Honolulu, the case fatality rate decreased from 30% in 1969–72 to 16% in 1985–88. A decline in case fatality may be due to changes in natural history, with fewer severe strokes, or to better medical management, or to better case ascertainment in the population, resulting in more mild stroke events being identified. The only population in which an increase in the case fatality rate was reported was Lithuania. Between the two time periods (1986–89 and 1990–93) the case fatality rate increased annually by 1.5% in men and by 1% in women.[8,31,32] The risk of death at 5 years was in the range 40–60%.

Changes in risk factor prevalence over time are one possible explanation for the change in stroke mortality rates. Risk factor change could directly influence incidence rates or indirectly change the case fatality rates by influencing the natural history of the disease.[29] A more likely explanation for the variations in case fatality rate over time is that the natural history of stroke is changing. Better treatment of hypertension, improved metabolic control of diabetes and antithrombotic therapy in patients at high risk for embolic strokes may not only reduce the incidence of stroke, but may perhaps also reduce the severity of the disease when it occurs.[25]

Wolfe and colleagues[33] demonstrated in southern England that the variation in the standardised mortality ratio for stroke in those aged under 75 years could be explained by variations in the incidence of stroke, case fatality being similar in the regions studied. The methodology developed by Wolfe and colleagues to explain the variations in mortality included population-based stroke registers in three geographical areas, recording all 'first in a lifetime' strokes and deaths within a 2-year period of the stroke. As part of the data collection, resource use information on admission to hospital, type of hospital bed used, use of brain imaging, length of stay and access to rehabilitation services were recorded. Collection of these data across centres enabled the study to identify variations in the resource inputs to care and inequities in service provision.

Similar methodologies have been used to examine the variations in death rates from bladder cancer. Walker and colleagues[34] set out to assess the individual contributions of incidence and case fatality to variations in bladder cancer mortality in southern England. They calculated the district standardised mortality ratios (SMRs) for bladder cancer using data from the local cancer registry and compared these with the standardised registration ratios, used as a measure of incidence, and survival hazard function. As severity at presentation is one determinant of case fatality, they also compared mortality with the standardised proportional hazards model to measure survival from diagnosis. Mortality from bladder cancer was significantly related to measurements of incidence, case fatality, and severity of presentation. They suggested that there is a need for further studies to investigate why some districts had high standardised registration ratios and risk of death. There may have been variation between districts with regard to the completeness of cancer registration and the accuracy of recording the stage of disease.

Treurniet and colleagues[35] have studied the association between regional variations in avoidable mortality and variation in disease incidence. For hypertensive and cerebrovascular disease there were significant regional variations in mortality. The variation in mortality was only partly explained by variations in incidence, being 34.6% for cerebrovascular disease and hypertension, and as low as 1% for appendicitis. In total, 60% of the variation in total cause-specific mortality was accounted for by in-hospital mortality. This is in contrast to a figure of 29% for cervical cancer. The study used data on discharge from hospital to estimate incidence, though this is likely to be an underestimate since not all cases are admitted to hospital. Although this study illustrated the possible associations between incidence and mortality using routine data, it was unable to explain the differences any further. Adjustment for confounders such as case severity would indicate whether the in-hospital mortality differences were real or merely reflected differences in case severity.

Other methods used to investigate the high mortality rates include confidential enquiries and audit. These can explicitly analyse the process and outcome of care compared with set standards, although for many published confidential enquiries the process of peer review may not be objective or standardised. Case–control studies have also been used to assess the contribution of various factors, such as hypertension control and stroke, to death.

Within the European Union-funded biomedical and health research initiatives, studies aimed at explaining such differences have been funded. Eurocare-2 aims to explain the reasons for the observed differences in cancer survival within Europe,[36] while for stroke the Biomed II stroke study, detailed in this book, was set up to explore the relationship between resource use, costs and outcome of different patterns of stroke care.

Interpreting variations in stroke management across countries

The impact of stroke on health services varies between countries. Studies in the UK have indicated that 55% of patients are admitted to hospital.[37] French studies suggest that different types of stroke may be treated in different hospitals, more severe strokes being treated in public hospital (70%), and milder strokes being treated in private clinics (20%) or at home.[38–40] Hospital services as well as primary and community care are fragmented and poorly tailored to stroke patients' needs. The MONICA study also found that the proportion of non-fatal stroke cases diagnosed and treated in the community ranged from 0% to 16% in 13 populations.[14] With the ageing population and potential for acute therapies for stroke, the proportion of hospital costs spent on stroke will increase. In addition to direct hospital costs, there will be direct costs related to long-term care of disabled survivors, and indirect costs relating to care.

There are considerable limitations to the use of routine data to answer questions about the service and financial impact of stroke. A gold-standard methodology would be to have population-based registers with follow-up of all patients documenting incidence, case severity, use of resources and their costs and outcome. Such studies are few and far between, and their cost-effectiveness is unclear. To date, no population-specific register data have been used in this way, and certainly no comparisons between centres have been attempted. However, interpretation of different data sets with a multitude of biases means that when variations are identified, it is difficult to determine whether these are true or artefactual. Official mortality data are readily available and therefore convenient. However, they rely on the accuracy of death certificates, which is questionable and only provides information about fatal cases of stroke, telling us nothing about the significant proportion of stroke patients who survive, many of them with major disability. Furthermore, without a knowledge of the accuracy of the diagnostic methods employed, they cannot tell us about the distribution of the different pathological types of stroke. Several possible explanations exist for the substantial differences in stroke mortality between countries, and its trends with time. For example, the apparent recent decline in stroke mortality in many Western countries may reflect either changes in diagnostic fashions and coding procedures, or a real decline that can be explained by changes in incidence and/or case fatality. The latter may depend on the distribution of pathological types, disease severity and management. A clearer, more complete picture can only be obtained by examining incidence and case fatality rates separately. If they are accurate, these measures allow more valid comparisons between countries, and may yield data that can be used to follow trends with time and assist in healthcare planning within communities.

Conclusion

The health service researcher can use several potential methodologies as listed below when investigating aspects of mortality in a defined geographical area or hospital setting:

- confidential enquiries into cases
- audit of care
- prospective studies using chronic disease registers (e.g. cancer, stroke)
- case–control studies.

The international literature demonstrates that there are unexplained variations in the impact of stroke, as for most of the major diseases. Studies of variations in incidence and mortality often fail to collect relevant data to interpret variations in the outcome of stroke, merely documenting the impact at one time point or at best over a short period of time.

The authors of this book are collaborators in two European Union Biomed Concerted Actions designed to begin to identify the reasons behind the variation in mortality from stroke between member states.

The objectives of the first Concerted Action (1993–95) were as follows:

- to maintain hospital- and community-based stroke registers for recording the care and outcome of stroke patients in nine centres in England, France, Italy, Germany, Portugal, Hungary and Poland
- to measure the resources used by each centre's treatment package for stroke patients (e.g. hospital/home care, level of rehabilitation support)
- to assess the cost of different packages of care and analyse the reasons for cost variations between centres (e.g. to determine whether they are due to differences in the price, type or volume of input)
- to compare packages of care in different centres in terms of resource use and outcome (i.e. mortality, disability, handicap and quality of life)
- to provide a framework which allows other European centres to assess the resource and cost implications of establishing desired treatment packages in their locality.

The second Concerted Action (1995–98) developed these themes further with additional centres in Finland, Denmark, Latvia, Lithuania, Russia and Austria. The specific aims were as follows:

- to quantify the resources and costs devoted to stroke care by primary, ambulatory, community and hospital services, and by patients and their carers
- to quantify the outcome of care in terms of mortality, impairment, disability and patient quality of life
- to quantify the relationship between patient outcomes and the resources and costs devoted to stroke care
- as a result, to develop protocols which describe how the overall resources devoted to stroke care can best be deployed so as to improve the range of patient outcomes
- in achieving these objectives, the project aimed to develop general methodologies for comparing across states the resources, costs and outcomes of stroke care which would be applicable to other common conditions
- to disseminate throughout participating centres across Europe techniques for measuring resources, costs and outcomes of stroke care and, as a consequence, to extend the research capabilities in these centres.

The subsequent chapters of this book will describe Concerted Action's attempts to answer these questions. The methodologies used, the results and the lessons learned will be discussed. The partners were chosen for Concerted Action for a variety of reasons, including the fact that they were known to the co-ordinator as being interested in stroke health services research, previous publications in the epidemiology/health service research of stroke, previous European research experience, or clinical expertise in the area of stroke. Although this is a case study of stroke, the authors will identify the issues and solutions that are applicable to chronic diseases in general that have a significant impact in Europe.

References

1 World Health Organisation (2000) *The World Health Report 2000. Health systems: improving performance.* World Health Organisation, Geneva.
2 Murray CJL and Lopez AD (1997) Mortality by cause for eight regions of the world: global burden of disease study. *Lancet.* **349**: 1269–76.
3 The Stroke Association (1998) *Stroke Care: reducing the burden of disease.* The Stroke Association, London.
4 Sarti C, Rastenyte D, Cepaitis Z and Tuomilehto J (2000) International trends in mortality from stroke. *Stroke.* **31**: 1588–601.
5 Wolfe CDA and Burney PGJ (1992) Is stroke mortality on the decline in England? *Am J Epidemiol.* **136**: 558–65.

6   Gillum RF and Sempos CT (1997) The end of the long-term decline in stroke mortality in the United States. *Stroke*. **28**: 1527–9.

7   Holland WW (1991) *European Community Atlas of Avoidable Death. Vol. 1* (2e). Oxford University Press, Oxford.

8   Schoenberg BS and Schulte BPM (1988) Cerebro-vascular disease: epidemiology and geopathology. In: PJ Vinken, GW Bruyn, HL Klawans and JF Toole (eds) *Vascular Diseases (Part 1)*. Elsevier Science, Amsterdam, 1–26.

9   WHO MONICA Project (prepared by P Thorvaldsen, K Kuulasmaa, AM Rajakangas, D Rastenyte, C Sarti and L Wilhelmsen) (1997) Stroke trends in the WHO MONICA Project. *Stroke*. **28**: 500–6.

10 Stegmayr B (1996) *Stroke in the community. Studies on risk factors, incidence, case fatality, severity and secular trends in the Northern Sweden MONICA Project with multinational comparisons*. Umea University Medical Dissertations, Umea.

11 WHO MONICA Project (prepared by P Thorvaldsen, K Asplund, K Kuulasmaa, AM Rajakangas and M Schroll) (1995) Stroke incidence, case fatality and mortality in the WHO MONICA Project. *Stroke*. **26**: 361–7.

12 Sudlow CLM and Warlow CP (1997) Comparable studies of the incidence of stroke and its pathological types. Results from an international collaboration. *Stroke*. **28**: 491–9.

13 Giroud M, Milan C, Beuriat P *et al.* (1991) Incidence and survival rates during a two-year period of intracerebral and subarachnoid haemorrhages, cortical infarcts, lacunes and transient ischaemic attacks: the Stroke Registry of Dijon 1985–1989. *Int J Epidemiol*. **20**: 892–9.

14 Asplund K, Bonita R, Kuulasmaa K *et al.* (1995) Multinational comparisons of stroke epidemiology. *Stroke*. **26**: 355–60.

15 Criqui MH and Ringal BVL (1994) Does diet or alcohol explain the French paradox? *Lancet*. **344**: 1719–23.

16 Thorvaldsen P, Asplund K, Kuulasmaa K, Rajakangas A and Schroll M for the WHO MONICA Project (1995) Stroke incidence, case fatality and mortality in the WHO MONICA Project. *Stroke*. **26**: 361–7.

17 Chen D, Roman GC, Wu GX *et al.* (1992) Stroke in China (Sino–MONICA-Beijing Study) 1984–1986. *Neuro-epidemiology*. **11**: 15–23.

18 Malmgrem R, Warlow C, Bamford J and Sandercock P (1987) Geographical and secular trends in stroke incidence. *Lancet*. **2**: 1196–200.

19 Tanaka H, Veda Y, Date C *et al.* (1981) Incidence of stroke in Shibata Japan: 1976–1978. *Stroke*. **12**: 460–6.

20 Sudlow CLM and Warlow CP (1996) Comparing stroke incidence worldwide. What makes studies comparable. *Stroke*. **27**: 550–58.

21   Brown RD, Whisnant JP, Sicks JD, O'Fallon WM and Wiebers DO (1996) Stroke incidence, prevalence and survival. Secular trends in Rochester, Minnesota, through 1989. *Stroke.* **27**: 373–80.

22   Truelsen T, Prescott E, Gronbaek M, Schnohr P, Boysen G (1997) Trends in stroke incidence. The Copenhagen City Heart Study. *Stroke.* **28**: 1903–7.

23   Tuomilehto J, Rastenyte D, Sivenius J *et al.* (1996) Ten-year trends in stroke incidence and mortality in the FIN-MONICA Stroke Study. *Stroke.* **27**: 825–32.

24   Bonita R, Broad JB and Beaglehole R (1993) Changes in stroke incidence and case fatality in Auckland, New Zealand, 1981–1991. *Lancet.* **342**: 1470–73.

25   Truelsen T *et al.* (1997) *op cit.*

26   Stegmayer B, Asplund K and Wester PO (1994) Trends in incidence, case fatality rate and severity of stroke in Northern Sweden, 1985–1991. *Stroke.* **25**: 1738–45.

27   Terent A (1988) Increasing incidence of stroke among Swedish women. *Stroke.* **19**: 598–603.

28   Tuomilehto J, Bonita R, Stewart A *et al.* (1990) Hypertension, cigarette smoking, and the decline in stroke incidence in eastern Finland. *Stroke.* **22**: 7–11.

29   Bonita R (1994) Epidemiological studies and the prevention of stroke. *Cerebrovasc Dis.* **4 (Supplement 1)**: 2–10.

30   Mackenbach JP, Bouvier-Colle MH and Jougla E (1990) Avoidable mortality and health services: a review of aggregate data studies. *J Epidemiol Commun Health.* **44**: 106–11.

31   Rastenyte D, Tuomilehto J, Sarti C, Cepaitis Z and Bluzhas J (1996) Trends in the incidence and mortality of stroke in Kaunas, Lithuania, 1986–1993. *Cerebrovasc Dis.* **6**: 13–20.

32   Rastenyte D, Cepaitis Z, Sarti C, Bluzhas J and Tuomilehto J (1995) Epidemiology of stroke in Kaunas, Lithuania: first results from the Kaunas stroke register. *Stroke.* **26**: 240–4.

33   Wolfe CDA, Taub N, Woodrow J *et al.* (1993) Does the incidence, severity or case fatality of stroke vary in southern England? *J Epidemiol Commun Health.* **47**: 144–8.

34   Walker A, Petruckevitch A, Bourne H and Burney P (1992) Contributions of incidence and case fatality to mortality from bladder cancer in the South Thames regions. *J Epidemiol Commun Health.* **46**: 387–9.

35   Treurniet HF, Looman CWN, van der Maas PJ and Mackenbach JP (1999) Variations in 'avoidable' mortality: a reflection of variations in incidence. *Int J Epidemiol.* **28**: 225–32.

36 Berrino F (1995) Eurocare-2. Cancer registries-based study on survival and care of cancer. In: A-E Baert *et al.* (eds) *European Union Biomedical and Health Research. The Biomed 1 Programme.* IOS Press, Amsterdam, 316–17.

37 Beech R, Ratcliffe M, Tilling K and Wolfe C (1996) Hospital services for stroke care. A European perspective. *Stroke.* **27**: 1958–64.

38 Giroud M, Lemesle M, Quantin C *et al.* (1997) A hospital-based and a population-based stroke registry yield different results: the experience in Dijon, France. *Neuro-epidemiology.* **16**: 15–21.

39 Giroud M, Lemesle M, Madinier G, Menassa M, Billiar TH and Dumas R (1998) Clinical patterns of acute stroke among the three health-care systems in France. *Eur J Neurol.* **5**: 463–7.

40 Bonita R, Stewart A and Beaglehole R (1990) International trends in stroke mortality: 1970–1985. *Stroke.* **21**: 989–92.

CHAPTER 2

Building workable data sets for health services research

Ruth Dundas, Daiva Rastenyte and Peter Heuschmann

Introduction

Chapter 1 identified the significant international and European variations in stroke incidence and outcome. The factors that drive these differences are likely to be complex, as they are affected by the age, sex and social structure of the populations, differences in risk factor profiles, differences in healthcare systems and the ways in which individual patients are treated. Some of the apparent variation may reflect problems with data collection. If the definitions of the variables across centres and countries being compared are open to interpretation, then systematic bias could be introduced.

This chapter addresses the issues of developing and implementing data sets for comparing stroke care services, which can be used in different clinical settings around Europe.

Factors that will be discussed in this chapter include the following:

- the choice of variables to be collected in order to answer the questions
- the feasibility of collecting these data
- the need to pilot questionnaires for validity and reliability
- the need for monitoring of data quality and the analysis of data.

Scope for the survey

A survey is a research technique used to gather information. Surveys are used in a wide range of disciplines (e.g. sociology, psychology, health services research and demography) to collect information on a wide range of subjects. It is a method of collecting a systematic set of data from many cases (patients or individuals), with the same variables collected for each patient or individual. The survey involves developing a research hypothesis, through questionnaire design to analyses and reporting of results. There are certain key requirements for a good survey which encompass all aspects of this process. These requirements are summarised by Fink.[1] As with any research method, before considering what data are to be collected, some thought should have gone into the aim of the survey and whether the objectives are actually measurable. Once the aims and objectives have been clarified, the study design should then be decided (e.g. randomised controlled trial, observational, cohort, cross-sectional, hospital based) and a sample selected. It is only when all of these requirements have been met that the stage of developing reliable and valid instruments for data collection is reached.

Principles of data collection

Types of variables

A discrete variable is a characteristic with at least two categories (e.g. sex is a variable with the two categories female and male), whereas a continuous variable has many categories (e.g. age). Each case will only feature in one category (a case cannot be both male and female) and each variable will encompass all categories (a case has to be either female or male and no other category). There are an infinite number of potential variables which are available to be collected for each study. However, once the main aims have been decided upon, these determine which variables need to be collected in order to answer the question. The explanatory (or independent) variables can be thought of as belonging to three different types:[2]

- essential to determine the effect on outcome (e.g. number of CT scans, amount of therapy input)
- potential confounding variables (e.g. age, sex, pre-stroke disability, pathological type of stroke), case mix (e.g. conscious level and continence at maximum impairment)
- variables of potential interest to secondary aims (e.g. risk factors for stroke, delay to admission).

Choosing the variables

The first process that needs to be completed when deciding which variables to choose is deciding the precise questions that the research is attempting to answer. If the research is unfocused this will result in a series of data items being collected that will not be used in the final analysis. It will give rise to difficult and unwieldy questionnaires, and the quality of data collection will probably be compromised. This is particularly important in multicentre, international studies where the qualifications and experience of data collectors may vary widely, and where the data are being collected by individuals as part of their routine clinical work. It is better to compromise on quantity and settle for quality.

An important consideration when deciding to collect data on a particular variable is how the variable will be used in the analysis. For instance, if the primary interest is in resource use (e.g. the numbers of patients receiving blood tests), then collecting data on the actual level of lipids in the blood in mmol/L is not necessary. All that is required is to establish whether a blood test was performed. It is a difficult aspect of any study to decide on appropriate variables to collect, as the tendency is to become very excited about the potential of the study and end up with a 15-page questionnaire with sections on detailed risk factors and diagnostic test results. This is not only tedious but may result in the questionnaire not being filled in completely as there will be too much information to collect, and important variables may become redundant and consequently have to be dropped from the analysis. It is much better to be ruthless and focus on fewer key variables, which will be collected in full for everyone.

Box 2.1   Choosing variables

- Decide on the question being addressed.
- Quality of data is more important than quantity.
- Only record a variable in a way that can be used for analysis.
- Categorise variables by using meaningful clinical groupings.

Avoiding errors

Davies and Smith[3] acknowledge that 'data processing is the least glamorous aspect of research', but they also point out that 'probably at no other stage is there a greater chance of a bad error being made. To avoid errors, checks and safeguards must be built into the system.' For example, in the World Health Organisation MONICA project,[4] all checks and cross-checks were performed by means of both manual checking and computer programs and conducted in both the collaborating centre and the data-processing (or organising) centre. Manual checks involved assurance that there were no blanks and everything was in a logical order. Special computer programs were created on the basis of a written algorithm that firstly described legal and illegal values for different variables, and secondly made logical consistency between codes assigned for different variables that were related between themselves. For example, the variable 'sex' can have only two possible values, such as '1' for males and '2' for females, so any other value, for example 3 or 4, will not be permitted. As an example of logical internal consistency, consider the internal relationship between the variable 'survival' and the variable 'date of death'. If we have a case of stroke which is known to be alive on the 28th day after the onset, 'survival' has to be coded as '1' (alive) and 'date of death' as 88/88/88 (not relevant for a case). If the computer program finds 'survival' coded as '2' (dead) and 'date of death' as 88/88/88, or 'sex' coded as '3', it generates an error correction form. This form contains all constraint violations and therefore they can be corrected.[4]

Once the variables have been chosen, the next step is to decide on how the information should be collected. A continuous variable can be categorised at a later stage, but not vice versa. The tendency is to use too few categories, which will mask potentially meaningful associations. If one is using categorical variables it is important to make sure that the categories are mutually exclusive and completely specify all of the possible answers.

Choosing the variables for the Biomed stroke studies

The objectives for the Biomed I study, which have already been outlined in Chapter 1, were as follows:

- to describe variations between centres in their treatment policies and the utilisation of resources (e.g. home/hospital care, level of physiotherapy support)
- to assess the costs of different packages of care and analyse the reasons for cost variations between centres
- to compare packages of care in the different countries in terms of outcome and resource use.

Representative clinicians and researchers from each of the participating centres met at the beginning of the study for two days to set the aims of the project and decide on the key variables that would be needed to answer the questions set. Although most of the participants in this meeting were physicians (neurologists, general physicians and geriatricians), the group was greatly helped by the presence of a public health physician, a statistician and an operational researcher. The domains for the questions are listed in Box 2.2. Some of the centres were already using core data sets or had existing stroke registers,[5-7] and these were used as a starting point for deciding the Biomed data-set variables. Left to themselves, many of the physicians would have included a large number of data items describing in great detail the impairments of the patients and their subsequent progress. Each item was considered individually, but only those considered to be absolutely essential for the research questions, and feasible for collection in each of the centres, were finally included. This led to a certain amount of dissatisfaction among some of the participants. However, it was made clear that each centre was of course free to conduct parallel research and include whatever extra items they needed for such research. The Biomed variables were in this sense a 'minimum data set' for stroke, on to which other items for data collection could be bolted.

Box 2.2   Domains for data collection

Core patient identification data

Pre-stroke: Living conditions and employment status
Disability using either Barthel or Rankin score (decided locally)
Risk factors
Medication

Current stroke: Date of stroke and admission
Type of bed to which admitted, and subsequent bed transfers
Date of discharge
Stroke severity data (e.g. conscious level (coma or non-coma), paralysis, continence, swallowing problem)
Stroke-specific diagnosis (e.g. infarction, haemorrhage)

Resources used: Investigations performed (e.g. brain imaging, carotid Dopplers, echocardiography)
Therapy provided (e.g. physiotherapy, occupational therapy, speech therapy)

Date of death/discharge

3-month data: Place of residence
Clinicial status – impairments and disabilities (Barthel or Rankin score as for pre-stroke)
Complications of stroke (e.g. pressure sores)
Use of rehabilitation
Use of investigations
Contacts with professionals

Collecting reliable data

Following the first meeting a manual was written giving definitions for each of the questions so as to provide as little leeway as possible for individual and idiosyncratic interpretation. The questionnaires were piloted in each of the centres, and a second meeting was held to review the data set. This process revealed some interesting and unforeseeable problems in international data collection. In most countries, 'Home alone' was taken to mean that the person was living alone as a single person. However, in some centres it was interpreted as including living with a spouse. Whether this reflects a wider difference in the meaning of marriage across cultures was not explored further.

The group met twice a year for the duration of the study and developed close working relationships that made robust discussion about the project both easy and enjoyable. The development and use of the core data set was a reiterative process that could not have been achieved with only one or two meetings, and would have been impossible if attempted at a distance.

We did not undertake an inter-rater reliability study, as the resources available were insufficient to add further to data collection. Such a study has been performed as part of the National Sentinel Audit for Stroke in the UK.[8] Using similar questions and a detailed manual to assist auditors, high kappa values were obtained (Gomperz et al., personal communication). However, where possible we did use validated reliable tools to collect the data. For example, the Barthel Index has been shown to be valid internationally and to be collectable at interview, by post and by telephone.[9,10]

The major areas where there were problems with data collection included clinical subtype information, quantification of therapy provision and clinical data at the 3- and 12-month follow-up. In countries where the health system sharply divides primary and secondary care, obtaining data after discharge from hospital was particularly laborious and time-consuming. In general, the data were collected from clinical notes or as a result of direct questioning of the patient and their relatives. In routine collection, all of these variables (e.g. blood pressure) are subject to inter- and intra-observer variation. Unfortunately, such possible bias was not assessed in this health services research project.

Biomed I

The major finding from Biomed I was the unexplained variation in length of stay in hospital and survival, as well as other differences in resource use. For this reason, an application was made for funding to expand the breadth of the study to explore longer-term management across health and social care sectors.

The objectives of Biomed II were as follows:

* to quantify the resources and costs devoted to stroke care by primary, ambulatory, community and hospital services and by patients and their carers
* to quantify the outcomes in terms of mortality, impairment disability and quality of life
* to quantify the relationship between patient outcomes and the resources and costs devoted to stroke care.

Much the same process was completed for this second project to decide on the data that needed to be collected, although on this occasion the group was larger and included several centres from Eastern Europe. Members of the group were experienced in working together and were more aware of the issues identified in the first project. The domains are similar to those in Biomed I, but are often covered in more detail (*see* Box 2.3). Copies of data collection sheets are provided on the accompanying website, www.radcliffe-oxford.com/stroke1. Because of the difficulties experienced in collecting longer-term data in Biomed I, centres were encouraged to study a smaller number of patients more thoroughly (i.e. for a shorter period of time), but with enough cases to make comparisons worthwhile.

Box 2.3   Domains for questions in Biomed II

Patient identification data
Demographic data
Pre-stroke: Living conditions
                                   Disability (either Barthel or Rankin
                                       score, decided locally)
                                   Risk factors for stroke
                                   Drug treatment
Time and date of onset: Time to admission
Use of resources: Bed type and subsequent transfers
                                   Use of investigations
                                   Use of surgery
                                   Acute treatments
                                   Enteral feeding
                                   Rehabilitation
                                                              Cont

---

Stroke severity:	Impairments
	Stroke diagnosis (clinical status using Bamford classification and pathological criteria)
Discharge destination	
Functional status at discharge	
3-month follow-up:	Use of resources and clinical status (impairment disability and handicap)
Two simple questions	Do you feel that you have made a complete recovery from your stroke?
	In the last 2 weeks has the patient required help from another person for everyday activities?

Box 2.4 Questionnaire design

- Choose words whose meanings cannot be misinterpreted.
- Discuss each question with the data collectors prior to starting the study.
- Pilot questionnaires in as many of the participating sites as possible.
- Choose questions that are likely to be feasible for responses by the population under study.
- Where possible, use questions that have been previously tested for reliability and validity.
- Train observers in the use of scales of outcome.

Principles of data collection for cross-national comparisons

The issue of meaning and justification for a particular variable is of the utmost importance when performing a cross-national comparison. For each variable, a painstaking process of translation and back-translation and discussion of meaning should be undertaken. A fundamental requirement of cross-national studies is that the phenomena being compared must actually be comparable. Terms, categories and methods must be standardised wherever possible. It is not literal equivalence that matters, but rather it is semantic and conceptual equivalence of the terms and categories that is necessary. A question is said to be semantically equivalent if it has the same meaning across all countries. If the responses to a question are shown to be indicators of the same concept across countries, then the question can be accepted as being conceptually equivalent. To standardise the methods, careful control of the data collection process is necessary. This may be problematic, as obviously the process is taking place in more than one country. Just as the research instruments have to be equivalent, so must the research procedures. This is achieved by developing a detailed protocol and translating it where necessary, together with appropriate training of observers. There are numerous sources of error in any survey conducted in one location,[11] and these are multiplied when a survey is conducted in more than one location. These sources of bias and error can be reduced if the established protocol is adhered to strictly. The procedure should be monitored by one overall co-ordinator who visits each of the participating countries. This co-ordinator should also provide the training for each research team.

Data entry

In the Biomed studies, as outlined above, regular meetings with participants, ownership of the questionnaire by all involved in the study, piloting of questions and development of a terminology manual all increased the likelihood of complete, accurate data collection across centres. When conducting a cross-national survey, the way in which the data are entered into the computer is important. Compatibility between all of the systems needs to be ensured. One effective way of achieving this is to develop a detailed codebook. Once the variables have been decided upon and the categories chosen, then a codebook is generated. The latter forms part of the manual and indicates where each variable is located in the data set along with the coding for individual questions. It may also contain information on what to do if two answers are checked for a question. Usually a blank questionnaire can serve as the codebook, but a separate codebook can be prepared. It is necessary to establish some rules about the way in which data are to be transferred. It is easiest for each centre to be responsible for their own data entry, so that the data are transferred to the co-ordinating centre electronically and not in paper format. Data should be sent in the format laid out in the codebook, and only the variables that are specified in the codebook should be sent. Occasionally a centre will be collecting the data for different purposes or as part of a larger study. Some variables will be collected that are not relevant to the cross-national study, and it is confusing and time-consuming for the co-ordinating centre to have to deal with these extraneous variables. A label which specifies the names of the data files should be clearly marked on the disk. In the WHO MONICA project, although most of the collaborating centres were collecting more data than was necessary for the core MONICA study, it was strongly recommended that only the core data should be extracted from the more extensive data set for transmission to the co-ordinating centre.[4]

The extraction of the core data is the most critical stage of the data transfer. In the MONICA study it was usually achieved by using a computer program.[4] Any errors in the core data induced by an erroneous program are systematic. Therefore special attention was paid to detecting all possible errors in the data extraction program. This included selecting a sample of records for which a data-transfer format was then filled in manually from the original data collection forms (including error corrections) by a qualified person. The sample size was at least 20 if the extraction consisted of only a selection of items from the local data set. However, if the value of a core data item was a combination of the values of one or several local data-set items, the correctness of such core data items was checked more carefully. In particular, a larger sample, at least for such items, was considered. The manually completed forms were then compared with the core data extracted by the computer. Before submitting data to the co-ordinating centre they should be checked for completeness, ensuring that all records are present, and that the data are correct and consistent. The data should be checked to ensure that they will not contain illegal values.

For the Biomed study, data completion was mainly performed by clinicians in the hospitals. This proved to be difficult in some instances, and was greatly helped by having a dedicated named data management person/ statistician with whom to liaise with at each centre. Each centre was responsible for its own data entry and was provided with a standardised database package, although some centres used their own package. The database package that was used for Biomed II was Epi Info. This is a word-processing, database and statistics program for public health, written by the Centers for Disease Control and Prevention, USA and the World Health Organisation, Switzerland (Epi Info is available as freeware from the Centers for Disease Control and Prevention website: http://www.cdc.gov/epiinfo/index.htm). There were a number of reasons why it was chosen. Epi Info is available as freeware, and all centres were able to run and use it. The co-ordinating centre wrote the entry program, with built-in checks. This meant that when the data were sent to the co-ordinating centre only some range checks and coding checks were required. Some centres used their own data-entry package, and their data were usually sent as a plain ASCII text file with an additional format statement and codebook. In order to create the data set for all of the centres, these data files had to be reformatted and recoded in the same way as the Biomed codebook. This can be a time-consuming exercise, since in some centres the coding for each variable had to be changed as they had coded YES = 1 and NO = 2, whereas in Biomed it was the other way round (i.e. NO = 1 and YES = 2).

Box 2.5   Data entry

- Collect the data in a form that is ready for direct entry into a computer.
- Develop a codebook.
- Make each centre responsible for its own data entry.
- Only use the core data set for entry to the central database.
- Develop systems for detecting data errors.
- Identify an individual who will be responsible for data entry in each centre.

Conclusions

Collection of large amounts of data from many centres in many countries is a difficult, time-consuming and expensive process. The key components involved are as follows:

- international data collection requires considerable resources
- collection of data on the process of care and outcome of stroke in different countries is feasible
- meetings to agree questions and questionnaire
- piloting data collection
- training of data-collection personnel
- development of a manual of terminology and agreed processes
- development of a computer program to ensure that illogical data are not entered.

Detail may have to be compromised in many instances for the sake of simplicity and accuracy. Nevertheless, this need not impede the overall research objectives. Time spent on careful questionnaire development is a worthwhile investment, focusing specifically on choosing valid and reliable questions that are essential for the study objectives. Equally important is the development of systems for full and accurate data collection and data entry.

The principal outcome measures that we used for both studies were the Barthel Index and mortality. For a complex, chronic disease such as stroke these are relatively crude outcome measures that may not cover some of the areas that matter to patients, such as mood and cognitive status, but they can be collected reliably by professionals with different levels of experience and in different cultural settings. There is evidence that the Barthel Index is correlated with many other outcome measures which are used for stroke. Therefore it may be used as a proxy for different outcome measures intended for the assessment of other domains.[12]

The participating centres were self-selected and do not claim to be representative of all hospitals in their countries. Hospital admission rates vary widely between countries, and therefore the patients studied represent only a subset of the stroke population. In order to address this issue, those European centres which are operating community stroke registers are now collaborating in further population studies addressing the issues posed in the Biomed programme. This cannot be done country-wide or continent-wide without substantial resources, so there still remains the problem of only a tiny proportion of all stroke patients being sampled for study.

Both Biomed I and Biomed II were successful collaborations, producing data that have proved of interest to many of those working in stroke care. They have shown that it is feasible to agree a data set between clinicians with widely differing backgrounds and perceptions about where the emphasis should lie in stroke care. The studies have shown that in many cases the data can be collected by busy clinicians without any additional resources. It is a strength of the study that many of the participating centres were not specialist stroke centres, and this is a finding that might be of relevance for others attempting to evaluate medical care in the settings where the majority of patients are treated.

The same principles of questionnaire design, data collection and collation are germane to most diseases, and most of the non-stroke data items discussed are relevant to all diseases studied in the variety of healthcare settings across Europe. Disease-specific variables can again be identified from previous international studies, and consensus among participants achieved in the studies being planned.

References

1   Fink A (1995) *How to Design Surveys. No. 5 in the survey kit.* Sage, Thousand Oaks, CA.

2   Singleton RA, Straits BC and Straits, MM (1993) *Approaches to Social Research* (2e). Oxford University Press, New York.

3   Davies JA and Smith TW (1992) *The NORC General Social Survey: a user's guide.* Sage, Newbury Park, CA.

4   Asplund K, Tuomilehto J, Stegmayr B, Wester P and Tunstall-Pedoe H (1988) Diagnostic criteria and quality control of the registration of

stroke events in the MONICA Project. *Acta Med Scand.* **728 (Supplement)**: 26–39.

5   Giroud M, Lemesle M, Quantin C *et al.* (1997) A hospital-based and a population-based stroke registry yield different results: the experience in Dijon, France. *Neuroepidemiology.* **16**: 15–21.

6   Stewart JA, Dundas R, Howard RS, Rudd AG and Wolfe CD (1999) Ethnic differences in incidence of stroke: prospective study with stroke register. *BMJ.* **318**: 967–71.

7   Thorvaldsen P, Asplund K, Kuulasmaa K, Rajakangas AM and Schvoll M (1995) Stroke incidence, case fatality and mortality in the WHO MONICA project. *Stroke.* **26**: 361–7.

8   Rudd AG, Irwin P, Rutledge Z *et al.* (1999) The National Sentinel Audit for Stroke: a tool for raising standards of care. *J R Coll Phys Lond.* **33**: 460–4.

9   Kornerbitensky N and Wood-Dauphinee S (1995) Barthel Index information elicited over the telephone – is it reliable? *Am J Phys Med Rehab.* **74**: 9–18.

10 Wolfe C, Taub N, Woodrow J and Burney P (1991) Assessment of scales of disability and handicap for stroke patients. *Stroke.* **22**: 1242–4.

11 Moser CA and Kalton G (1971) *Survey Methods in Social Investigation* (2e). Dartmouth Publishing, Aldershot.

12 Wilkinson PR, Wolfe CDA, Warburton FG *et al.* (1997) Longer-term quality of life and outcome in stroke patients: is the Barthel Index alone an adequate measure of outcome? *Qual Health Care.* **6**: 125–30.

CHAPTER 3

Population disease registers

Peter Kolominsky, Mehool Patel,
Danuta Ryglewicz and Maurice Giroud

Introduction

A great deal of interest has been shown internationally in the development of disease management programmes as a means of improving the overall standard of care delivered to patients with chronic diseases. Part of this initiative has been the attention given to population-based disease-specific patient registers which have been recognised by many health service professionals as being a prerequisite for improving the quality of healthcare delivered. This recognition is despite the lack of systematically reviewed research evidence for their use. The development of registries can be traced back as far as 1086 to the preparation of England's *Domesday Book*.[1] In the field of stroke there has been a proliferation of population-based registries during the past 20 years.

Measurement of the overall health status of the population is an important public health issue. Such measurements that quantify the impact of disease are important in the context of clinical audit activities and healthcare decision making. The measurements can include prevalence rates, incidence rates, different measures of mortality and the number of cases of different diseases. The process of measuring the burden of illness must include indicators that fully reflect the effects of disease on society.

Mortality data only reflect one aspect of health, and are of limited value with regard to conditions that are rarely fatal, such as the most disabling chronic diseases, including stroke, dementia and degenerative joint diseases.

Measures of morbidity reflect another important aspect of the burden of illness. In addition, increasing attention is being given to measurement of the consequences of disease (i.e. impairment, disability and handicap).

Most hospital-based studies assessing outcome of chronic disabling diseases have been restricted to selected patients, such as those admitted to hospital or those referred for rehabilitation. A major disadvantage of such studies concerns the various forms of selection bias which may lead to a distortion of the true clinical course and prognosis. The variable case mix of hospital-based studies often limits the extent to which the information obtained may be extrapolated to other groups of patients. A comprehensive and sustainable picture of the disease outcome requires the inclusion of severely ill patients who are not admitted to hospital, as well as those with mild manifestation of the disease who are not admitted to hospital for rehabilitation – hence the concept of a population-based disease register (PDR) ascertaining all cases of a condition. To achieve complete case ascertainment, the PDR has to be truly population-based, although many registers are not so, merely listing cases presenting to or known by services (e.g. some stroke registers are solely based on stroke seen within acute hospitals, with the assumption that no cases remain at home). Registers that are not population based have considerable limitations in epidemiological terms, since they lack a reliable denominator, thus precluding, for example, the calculation of incidence rates. They are also unable to address issues of access to hospital care, as non-admitted patients are not registered and access is a key component of quality.

This chapter will address the following topics:

• the advantages and disadvantages of PDRs
• the use of PDRs for evaluation of outcome and quality
• characteristics of PDRs
• examples of PDRs.

Definition

Of the various definitions of a population-based register that have been documented, the most appropriate one is *'a database of identifiable persons containing a clearly defined set of health and demographic data collected for a specific public health purpose'*.[2]

Other definitions include the following:

• a list of people whose inclusion is predicated by their having a particular attribute (e.g. stroke)
• a file of documents containing uniform information about individual persons, collected in a systematic and comprehensive way in order to serve a predetermined purpose.[3]
• a system of recording frequently used in the general field of public health, which serves as a device for the administration of programmes concerned with the long-term care, follow-up or observation of individual cases.[4]

Registers may be either action or information registers, the former playing a part in the delivery of healthcare to individuals (e.g. genetic registers), and the latter containing information for planning of research (e.g. cancer registers).

Advantages

Impact of illness

Population-based registers serve as valuable tools for epidemiological studies of diseases. They can collect the data that help to quantify the impact of disease, such as incidence, prevalence and recurrence rates, and natural history, including rates of survival, morbidity and disability, as well as the number of cases of different diseases. All of the limitations of hospital-based studies are overcome if population-based registers are employed.

To reap the full benefits of registers in terms of these measurements, it is essential to have a system of active and regular follow-up. This will ensure as much as possible the quality of the data and thus the accuracy of the estimates. Depending on the primary focus of the data collection, certain data items will be pursued more actively. For example, if incidence is the focus, active notification from all sources is required, whereas if longer-term prevalence is the focus, complete follow-up over time is required.

Planning of healthcare delivery systems

Data from population registers can be used to monitor disease outcome accurately and thereby secure, through the resources available, the maximum improvement in the physical and mental health of individuals with that disease. Information from registers can facilitate the delivery of targeted, evidence-based and cost-effective specialist care. This would be likely to improve local arrangements for the provision of care, ensure the appropriate levels of provision and enable the delivered care to be reviewed at both general practice and health authority levels.[5] The complex issues of equity of access to care can also be addressed using data from registers as a starting point.

Registers facilitate the aggregation and analysis of comparable data to enable comparisons to be made over time in primary and secondary care, and to assist health authorities with their strategic planning.[5] They also enable healthcare planners within a health authority to develop strategic policies for chronic disease management. Registers may be linked to data generated by clinical management systems and thus enable, for example, outpatient management and planning, contribution to clinical follow-up and assessment of treatment. Achievement of these objectives would probably result in improvements in clinical outcomes. To date there are no good examples of PDRs being used for this purpose.

Audit and training

Registers offer opportunities to collect and present data relevant to clinical audit, service evaluation and needs assessment, all of which are of increasing importance in quality assurance in different programmes. There are hospital-based data-collection systems for stroke in several countries in Europe which are used to compare clinical and health service data between centres (e.g. Bavaria, England and Wales, and Sweden). Registers can also potentially provide an important resource for teaching and training of clinical and other staff.

Clinical research

Registers provide a rich source for identifying prevalent or incident cases for further studies, such as case–control or intervention studies exploring disease determinants and therapeutic modifiers. They are also valuable for generating hypotheses from the observational data that they provide. PDRs reduce the problems of selection bias that can occur in such studies based on clinical series. Linkage with other data sources or registers is particularly valuable in developing analytical studies to identify and investigate determinants of disease. For example, linkage of the NHS Central Registry and the National Cancer Registry with occupational and other records has proved particularly valuable in this respect. Thus registers can assist in research by providing an end-point for prospective studies.

Evaluation of outcome and quality assessment

The systematic use of epidemiological principles and methods such as population-based disease registers for the evaluation of healthcare services is a relatively new development. The ultimate goal is to develop a rational process for setting priorities and allocating scarce healthcare resources. Because of the limited resources available for healthcare in all countries, choices have to be made between alternative strategies for improving health. Registers can potentially enable the assessment of access to care and intervention, and form a basis for assessment of standards of care against agreed guidelines for practice.

In summary, there is the potential for PDRs to be central to the following:

- measurement or assessment of the impact of illness
- identification of the causes of illness
- measurement of the effectiveness of different interventions in the population
- assessment of their efficiency in terms of resources used
- implementation of interventions
- monitoring of healthcare access and the process of healthcare in different settings
- estimation of the relationship between outcomes, such as impairment and disability with survival.

Is a population-based register required?

Given the long-term commitment of resources associated with PDRs and limited public health funding, proposals for any new registers should be carefully considered before being funded. There are several issues and questions that need to be addressed when determining whether a register is warranted, as illustrated in Box 3.1.

Box 3.1   Issues to be addressed when determining whether a register is appropriate[2]

Evaluation of the stated purpose
There must be a clear statement of purpose for every register proposal. This purpose should be evaluated to determine what health problem(s) the information can solve, or facilitate solving, and whether these problems should be pursued.

Consideration of existing alternative data sources
Existing data sources should be reviewed carefully before implementing a new register, in order to prevent the creation of a register that would collect information which is already available. PDRs should be compared with other types of registers such as hospital-based or GP-based registers, which may not be as exhaustive as population-based

Cont

---

ones, but may be cheaper, more practical and large enough to answer the questions for which the new register is being proposed.

Assessment of the practical feasibility of the register
Registers should only be implemented if there is a reasonable expectation that they can achieve their goals.
   Issues to be considered include the following:

- Would case ascertainment be too costly or invasive?
- Would the number of subjects included be adequate to obtain useful information?
- Would the level of reporting be reliably high?
- How co-operative would the sources of referral (e.g. general practitioners) be?
- Is the data set simple and agreed by all parties?
- Is the population size well estimated?

Likelihood of sufficient start-up and long-term funding
Cost is the foremost problem in initiating and running any register. Funds are required not only for data collection and processing tasks, but also for quality control, data analysis, interpretation and dissemination of important findings to relevant professional groups. The operation of a register requires a long-term commitment.

Evaluation of the cost-effectiveness of the register
The potential clinical benefits of a proposed register should be weighed against the costs of the register.

- Is it likely to improve clinical outcome?
- Will it assist the strategic planning of the service?

Factors that might be considered when determining the public health impact of the information that a register can provide include the total number of cases, incidence and prevalence, access to care, indices of severity (e.g. case fatality ratio), overall mortality rate, medical costs, indices of disability or lost productivity, indices of premature mortality (e.g. years of potential life lost), preventability and expected benefit of registry-provided information in reducing morbidity and mortality.

Should the register be disease-specific or generic?

Characteristics of a good register

What are the main features of a successful, efficient and effective register? Twelve factors, which are outlined below, are critical to successful development of the new register.

1   An implementation plan

An implementation plan addressing the following issues should be devised:

- development of a time-line
- discussion of the registry with relevant healthcare professionals
- identifying (or hiring) and training of register personnel
- estimating register size (prevalence, incidence) and projecting the duration of the register
- identifying sources of data and case ascertainment
- developing and organising systems for case finding
- obtaining hardware, software and data-processing packages
- development of a quality-control system.

2   Adequate documentation

Documentation should include who will operate the register, a description of the inclusion and exclusion criteria, definition of data sources, collection, editing and entry procedures, protocols for matching to other data sources, data-processing procedures, analyses that will be routinely conducted, confidentiality guidelines and access procedures. These procedures will ensure that all staff are working to the same objectives, identifying appropriate cases and documenting the relevant data. Such procedures make handover to new register staff more efficient, and they also form the basis for the methodology of the register in any publications that are produced using the data.

3   Quality-control procedures

Completeness, validity and timeliness are the three goals that help to determine the quality of the data in any register. Completeness is defined as the proportion of cases in the target population that appear in the register. Validity is the percentage of cases in the registry with a given characteristic (e.g. sex, stroke type) that 'truly' have this attribute. Timeliness may be important in those registers that identify individuals who need critical and rapid services (e.g. those with infectious diseases). Principles that are likely to ensure quality control include the following.

- Build quality into the system rather than adding it later. By having explicit quality-control procedures in a manual, and with regular audit of these procedures as outlined here, the quality is maintained throughout the data-collection period.
- A person should be responsible for quality control at every level.
- Explicit standards and procedures for evaluating the system regularly should be present.
- A feedback loop should be incorporated into the system to inform data handlers of errors. This will include a senior member of the register staff reviewing each data set before it is entered into the computer and identifying data items that are missing, out of range or inconsistent.

4   Case definition

Inclusion and exclusion criteria should be clear and unambiguous to allow consistent decisions to be made about inclusion across the range of potential cases that arise (e.g. definition of stroke, geographical limits of the register).

5   Case-finding (ascertainment) procedures

Case ascertainment refers to the methods and sources that are used to locate individuals who should be included in the register. A high level of case ascertainment must be achieved for a register to be useful. Active case-ascertainment systems use registry staff to actively locate individuals who are to be included in the register. Passive systems rely on physicians and other healthcare workers to report cases to the registry staff. Usually a combination of the two is employed. Multiple sources are usually used to increase the likelihood of case finding, although this does raise costs. Case reporting could be at the request of the registry, by specific legislative mandate or by administrative rules directed by a legislative mandate. When reporting is required by law, compliance is likely to be better.

6   Effective notification and backup systems

There should be effective notification systems to ensure that the maximum number of cases in the study area is registered. There should also be efficient and multiple backup systems to capture 'missed' cases.

7 Commitment from local data providers and registry staff

For a register to be successful, it is vital that the providers of data for the register are committed and motivated. Medical practitioners such as hospital consultants and general practitioners who will be the main sources of data need to be regularly updated on the register in order to keep them interested and motivated with regard to it. Any information that may be useful to them or to the local health services should be regularly disseminated to help to generate and maintain their interest and collaboration. The register staff should be equally enthusiastic and committed to their work, which requires incentives such as the writing of reports and publication of papers.

8 Determination of data elements

The golden rule of determining data elements is to keep it simple. This lowers cost, increases compliance, and reduces the time taken to get the data into the system. Although it is desirable to avoid collecting unnecessary data, it is also important to ensure that all of the essential data elements are collected from the inception of the register. Changing data elements over time increases the likelihood of confusion and introduction of errors into the data set, as well as limiting the usefulness of the register outputs. Data elements should all be clearly defined to facilitate consistency and data sharing. A major part of the task of data definition is the development of a coding scheme for categorical variables. Although this may sound simple, there are generally exceptions that need to be handled appropriately. Piloting the data-collection system is the best way to locate ambiguities that do not fit into the predefined categories.

9 Data collection and processing procedures

Data collection and processing procedures consume a major part of the resources required to run a register. Two issues that need to be addressed are the choice of data collection and entry methods, and implementation of data verification and editing procedures.

10 Data-access policy and confidentiality

The ability to access information in an efficient, flexible and timely manner is a key element of the success of a register. However, it is imperative to safeguard the confidentiality of the information in the registry. In addition to the ethical and legal implications of maintaining confidentiality, case ascertainment and data collection would be greatly compromised if the individuals supplying the information were not confident that it would be protected. Ethical permission to set up registers will be required from local ethics committees, and the law for this varies between countries. It is necessary to ensure that whenever a new objective is proposed for a register, the ethics committee approves the changes to data collection.

11 Data comparability

Data should be collected in ways that will make comparison with data from other registers possible. This is an important consideration for a successful register, given the increasing importance of national and international collaboration in clinical research.

12 Framework for dissemination of register data and findings

There should be plans and resources available for dissemination of the register findings to relevant professional groups. This brings the rationale for the register back into the discussion. There should be explicit objectives for data collection which will hopefully be asking relevant questions for research or health service planning and delivery.

Examples of population-based stroke registers

The importance of good incidence studies in stroke was clearly described by Malmgren and colleagues in 1987 [6] and brought up to date in 1996 by Sudlow and Warlow,[7] whose key criteria for comparable studies of stroke incidence are listed in Box 3.2.

Aspects of the epidemiology of stroke have already been discussed in Chapter 1, and here examples of stroke registers in Europe will be discussed. Several large population-based stroke registers have been set up covering many Eastern and Western European countries over the past 25 years. These registers have helped to improve out understanding of the disease and the variations in outcome across different parts of Europe.

Registers from Eastern European centres include those implemented in Estonia (1991–93),[8] Lithuania (1995),[9] USSR,[10] East Germany[11] and Poland

Box 3.2   Core criteria for a comparable study of stroke incidence

Standard definitions
WHO definition
First-in-a-lifetime stroke

Standard methods
Complete, community-based case ascertainment based on multiple overlapping sources
Prospective study design, ideally with 'hot pursuit of cases'
Large, well-defined, stable population
Reliable method for estimating denominator by sociodemographic groups (e.g. age, sex, social class)

Standard data presentation
Whole years of data
Not more than 5 years of data aggregated together
Data for men and women presented separately
Includes ages up to and above 85 years if possible
Standard mid-decade age bands used in publications
Unpublished 5-year age bands available for comparison with other studies
Presentation of 95% confidence intervals around incidence rates

(Warsaw Stroke Registry – WSR).[12] There are a number of examples of Western European studies. In Denmark, the Copenhagen City Heart Study[13] comprises 19 698 subjects who have been followed since 1976. In Italy, the SEPIVAC study[14] was conducted between 1986 and 1989 to determine the incidence and outcome of both transient ischaemic attack (TIA) and strokes. In Sweden, STROMA[15] was started in 1989, covering the city of Malmo. In France, there has been a stroke registry since 1985 in Dijon,[16] covering a population of 140 000. In England, the Oxfordshire Community Stroke Project (OCSP)[17] ran from 1981 to 1986. There are several ongoing registers in Europe, including those in Dijon, France,[16] in south London[18] and in Erlangen, Germany.[19]

The largest epidemiological study of heart disease and stroke in younger people undertaken to date has been the MONICA project[20] (WHO Monitoring Trends and Determinants in Cardiovascular Disease). The stroke study encompassed 21 centres in 11 countries, covering a population of 2.9 million. The MONICA study showed considerable variation between countries in the age-standardised incidence rates per 100 000 in those aged

35–64 years. It was high in Finland (247–351 in men and 105–173 in women) and Russia (241–388 in men and 121–312 in women), moderate in Poland (184 in men and 90 in women), and low in Italy (124 in men and 61 in women) and Sweden (137 in men and 69 in women).

A good example of effective comparability and linkage with other registers is the European Registers of Stroke (EROS) network.[21] In 1997, three ongoing population-based stroke registers established the EROS network, which aimed to start a European Union stroke register. The data collected would reflect the impact of stroke across member states and describe variations which might be attributed to the different healthcare systems and specific attitudes towards management of stroke patients. These registers were the Dijon Stroke Register in France (started in 1985), the South London Stroke Register in England (started in 1995) and the Erlangen Stroke Project in Bavaria, Germany (started in 1994). These three registers agreed on a 'common methodological register language' with specific features and standards, including a high level of case ascertainment, clear case definitions, clear inclusion as well as exclusion criteria, uniform data collection, effective backup systems to capture 'missed' cases, quality-management systems to maintain data quality and completeness, and co-operation between local data providers. Examples of the data-collection sheets used in the South London Stroke Register can be found on the accompanying website, www.radcliffe-oxford.com/stroke2.

The EROS network has estimated the impact of stroke in specific regions of Europe. The European standardised incidence rate per 1000 was 1.19, ranging from 1.01 in Dijon to 1.23 in London and 1.36 in Erlangen ($p < 0.005$)

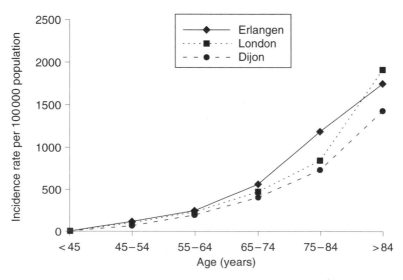

Figure 3.1 Age-specific incidence rates per 100 000 population.[21]

(*see* Figure 3.1). In all three EROS registers there were significantly increased rates in men, and an increase with age. In London, there were significant differences between Caucasian and black populations, with rates of 1.11/1000 and 2.68/1000, respectively. The overall case fatality rate was 35%, ranging from 27% in Dijon to 41% in London ($p < 0.001$), adjusted for age, sex and subtype.

Conclusions

This chapter has outlined the advantages of population-based registers for any disease for addressing a range of issues relating to the impact of and service provision for chronic diseases. The methods that need to be employed and the problems associated with maintaining a high-quality, relevant register are discussed. In terms of addressing the objectives outlined in Chapter 1, PDRs are an ideal vehicle, but would be required in many centres to address European issues. As such they are perhaps impractical, and other methods need to be explored as outlined elsewhere in this book.

There are considerable benefits to be derived from developing PDRs although the alternatives and cost-effectiveness both need to be considered. The benefits include the following:

- measurement or assessment of the impact of illness
- identification of the causes of illness
- measurement of the effectiveness of different interventions in the population
- assessment of the efficiency of those interventions in terms of resources used
- implementation of interventions
- monitoring of healthcare access and the process of healthcare in different settings
- estimation of the relationship between outcomes, such as impairment and disability with survival.

Developing and maintaining registers requires a thorough, standardised set of guidelines for case ascertainment, recording of data items, confidentiality and standard methods of data presentation.

References

1   Weddell JM (1973) Registers and registries: a review. *Int J Epidemiol.* **2**: 221–8.

2 Solomon DJ, Henry RC, Hogan JG *et al.* (1991) Evaluation and implementation of public health registries. *Pub Health Rep.* **106**: 142–50.

3 Brooke EM (1974) *The Current and Future use of Registers in Health Information Systems.* World Health Organisation, Geneva.

4 Bellows MT (1949) Case Registers. *Pub Health Rep.* **64**: 1148–58.

5 Dawson A (1996) *Chronic Disease Management Registers.* HMSO, London.

6 Malmgren R, Warlow C, Bamford J and Sandercock P (1987) Geographical and secular trends in stroke incidence. *Lancet.* **2**: 1196–200.

7 Sudlow CLM and Warlow C (1996) Comparing stroke incidence worldwide. What makes studies comparable? *Stroke.* **27**: 550–8.

8 Korv J, Roose M and Kaasik AE (1996) Changed incidence and case-fatality rates of first-ever stroke between 1970 and 1993 in Tartu, Estonia. *Stroke.* **27**: 199–203.

9 Rastenyte D, Cepaitis Z, Sarti C *et al.* (1995) Epidemiology of stroke in Kaunas, Lithuania: first results from the Kaunas stroke register. *Stroke.* **26**: 240–4.

10 Scmidt EV, Smirnov VE and Ryabova VS (1988) Results of the seven-year prospective study of stroke patients. *Stroke.* **9**: 942–9.

11 Eisenblatter D, Heinemann L and Claben E (1995) Community-based stroke incidence trends from the 1970s through the 1980s in East Germany. *Stroke.* **26**: 919–23.

12 Czlonkowska A, Ryglewicz D, Wessbein T *et al.* (1994) Prospective community-based study of stroke in Warsaw, Poland. *Stroke.* **25**: 547–51.

13 Truelsen T, Prescott E, Gronbaek M *et al.* (1997) Trends in stroke incidence. The Copenhagen City Heart Study. *Stroke.* **28**: 1903–7.

14 Caputo N, Chiurulla C, Scaroni R and Signorini E (1991) A community-based study of incidence, risk factors and outcome of transient ischaemic attacks in Umbria, Italy: the SEPIVAC study. *J Neurol.* **238**: 87–90.

15 Jerntorp P and Berglund G (1992) Stroke registry in Malmo, Sweden. *Stroke.* **23**: 357–61.

16 Giroud M, Beuriat P, Vion P *et al.* (1989) Stroke in a French prospective population study. *Neuroepidemiology.* **8**: 97–104.

17 Bamford J, Sandercock P, Dennis M *et al.* A prospective study of acute cerebrovascular disease in the community: the Oxfordshire Community Stroke Project 1981–1986. 1. Methodology, demography and incident cases of first-ever stroke. *J Neurol Neurosurg Psychiatry.* **51**: 1373–80.

18 Stewart J, Dundas R, Howard RS, Rudd AG and Wolfe CDA (1999) Ethnic differences in incidence of stroke: prospective study with stroke register. *BMJ.* **318**: 967–71.

19 Kolominsky-Rabas P, Sarti C, Heuschmann PU *et al.* (1998) A prospective community-based study of stroke in Germany. The Erlangen

Stroke Project (ESPro): incidence and case fatality at 1, 3 and 12 months. *Stroke.* **29**: 2501–6.

20 WHO MONICA Project (prepared by P Thorvaldsen, K Asplund, K Kuulasmaa *et al.*) Stroke incidence, case fatality and mortality in the WHO MONICA Project. *Stroke.* **26**: 361–7.

21 Wolfe CDA, Giroud M, Kolominsky-Rabas P *et al.* (2000) Variation in the incidence and survival of stroke in three areas of Europe. *Stroke.* **31**: 2074–9.

CHAPTER 4

The organisation of care: documenting services in different settings

Christopher McKevitt, Matias Torrent and Anthony Rudd

Introduction: the problem of unexplained variations in outcome

Studies evaluating health services typically use patient-based indicators, such as morbidity or mortality, to assess quality of care or efficacy of treatment. However, as earlier chapters have argued, interpreting such outcomes is not straightforward. A standard way of improving the interpretability of these data is to control for case mix, since differences in the characteristics of study populations – including age, gender and disease severity – can confound the results. Crude case-mix adjustment using merely age and sex is inadequate, as was demonstrated by a study of the effects of introducing a stroke unit in Scotland.[1] Unadjusted data clearly showed the benefits of stroke-unit care, and the effects were less marked but still significant when age and sex were taken into account. However, all differences in mortality and morbidity were eliminated when adjustment was made for case-severity measures, including incontinence in the first week, coma, motor impairment and social class.

This chapter will address the following topics:

- the problems of measuring outcome of care
- the problems of measuring the process of care
- the problems of measuring the structure of care and the context of health-care in the local setting
- the way in which these issues were tackled in the European Stroke Biomed Programme.

Measuring the outcome of care

A number of studies comparing outcomes across centres have demonstrated that differences in patient characteristics alone do not explain important differences in outcome. For example, the Biomed I study of hospital care for stroke patients in 12 European centres found significant differences in mortality and disability which were not explained by differences in case mix or service use (*see* Chapter 6 and Wolfe *et al.*[2]) An international meta-analysis of trials comparing organised inpatient (stroke unit) care with conventional care concluded that stroke units reduce stroke-related deaths and dependency in survivors.[3] Yet without more detailed information about the processes of care in stroke units, the authors could only speculate about how this model of care leads to improved results. Commenting on the variations in outcome in the International Stroke Trial, Signorini *et al.*[4] suggested that these might reflect the effect of confounding variables, or they might be the result of bias introduced by cross-cultural variations in definitions and reporting. Similarly, a number of multicentre outcome studies have shown that patient characteristics alone do not explain variations in the provision of care, including rates of hospitalisation and inpatient and outpatient rehabilitation.[5] For example, rates of admission to hospital as well as patterns of diagnosis and mortality are influenced by the distance from the patient's home to the hospital.[6] In another study covering 151 metropolitan areas in the USA, patient variables did not account for more than one-third of the variation in access to rehabilitation therapies following stroke.[7] There is no universally accepted system for defining factors influencing outcome that are patient related rather than treatment related. Although some attempts have been made to produce core data sets,[8] until these are systematically used for all studies of outcome, doubts will remain about the validity of comparison of data obtained from different clinical settings.

Measuring the process of care

These problems of interpreting the findings of outcome studies suggest a need for greater attention to be focused on the settings and structures of healthcare delivery. Therefore another strategy is to collect measures of processes of care in addition to patient outcomes. It has been suggested that measures such as length of stay in hospital provide indicators which are more easily measured and interpreted. Long and Fairfield[9] have proposed that evaluation of the effectiveness of services in fact requires monitoring of *both* process and outcomes. Here again there are some difficulties. Mackenbach *et al.*[10] considered the contribution of healthcare inputs to rates of avoidable mortality. In a review paper they concluded that studies investigating geographical variations in avoidable mortality may show a weak and inconsistent association with the provision of healthcare resources. However, one explanation for this finding may be that rather crude measures of the use of health services were employed in those studies (e.g. numbers of healthcare staff). It is possible that the way in which this supply is made to conform to quality standards and made accessible to the population is more important for the prevention of 'avoidable' deaths than the level of supply *per se*, and that these factors vary across regions independently of the level of supply. This would imply that a validation of avoidable mortality rates as indicators of the effectiveness of healthcare services should make use of measures of more specific aspects of healthcare delivery.[10] Treurniet *et al.*[11] investigated the value of including incidence data in studies of avoidable mortality variations, and argued that although this represents a step forward, further progress might be achieved by linking the approach of medical audit to descriptions of mortality variations.

The largest survey of the process of care for stroke patients in the UK was the National Sentinel Audit for Stroke.[12] Using a tool developed by an expert committee of professionals and patient and carer groups, and based wherever possible on evidence linking process to outcome, 80% of acute hospitals in England, Wales and Northern Ireland participated in the audit, contributing data on nearly 7000 patients. The results, despite the fact that they showed many areas of poor quality of care, were accepted by the participating clinicians and managers as being valid and representative of the service being provided. With only 40 patients being studied for each hospital, outcome data would have had little chance of being statistically useful for the comparison of services. For example, if pressure sore incidence was to be used as an adverse outcome measure, because of its relative rarity, 1240 patients in each hospital/time period would be needed to detect a change in incidence from 2% to 4% with 80% power and 95% confidence.

Measuring the structure of care

Even easier than audit of the process of care is audit of the structure and organisation of care within institutions. This defines what services and skills are available for the management of patients, but not necessarily what treatment patients actually receive. The Scottish Stroke Services Audit used this alone to define the standards of care.[13] It was also a component of the National Sentinel Audit for Stroke Care.[12] There was a moderate correlation (correlation coefficient $= 0.47$) between the audits of organisation and process (unpublished data).

Box 4.1

Measurement of process as a proxy for outcome avoids the need for case-mix adjustment, and it is immediately obvious what needs to be done to improve a service when the process is directly linked to outcome. The problem with the use of process measures arises in the many areas of clinical practice where there is no proven link between the process of care and the outcome. In such cases the outcome would need to be measured.

Where comparisons of service delivery across different countries are being made, as is increasingly the case, data collection and interpretation are further complicated by differences in the way in which healthcare services are delivered in different states. Such differences are assumed to be accounted for by the use of standardised process and outcome indicators, but the persistence of unexplained variations in outcome suggests a need to consider whether like is indeed being compared with like, and to examine whether new indicators should be measured. Standard indicators may not be sufficient to answer particular questions. Studies investigating methods of funding care[14] or the impact of physician type on process and outcomes[15] have necessarily included the relevant additional variables. Accounting for differences may therefore require the identification of further process indicators for inclusion in the analyses of outcomes.

Thus moving from evidence of variations in outcome to explaining how those variations arise may require additional information, including an understanding of economic, political and social processes which might influence, for example, decisions about 'appropriate' lengths of stay in hospital. Aiken and colleagues[16] have highlighted the importance of investigating how the structure and organisation of hospitals affect patient outcomes. From an anthropological perspective, Good[17] has drawn attention to local medical cultures which, albeit in a complex and shifting relationship with international standards of biomedical practice, influence the care which is available in particular settings. However, there has been little consideration of how such information should be collected. Ethnographic and observational methods appear to be appropriate, but can be time-consuming and costly. Despite a growing acceptance of qualitative methods in health research,[18] they are not normally integrated into international comparative studies of healthcare services and outcomes.

This chapter will illustrate the approach taken in the Biomed II study of stroke care and outcomes to address the problems identified.

Box 4.2   Why collect information about the structure of services?

Structures and processes of care vary from one locality to the next, particularly when cross-national comparisons are being made. Such information is needed to consider the usefulness of the indicators being used, and to interpret the results of quantitative data.

The Biomed II study problem

The participating centres in the Biomed II stroke study included centres in the Mediterranean countries and in Scandinavia, as well as centres in Western and Eastern Europe. Across Europe, healthcare and social care systems have developed in a variety of ways, with different methods of funding and different structures for the delivery of services. A number of descriptive accounts of different health and social care systems are available.[19,20] In addition to differences in the ways in which healthcare is funded and provided, there are important differences in culture, history, political systems and economic context, all of which may have an impact on the organisation and delivery of health, as well as the population's need for healthcare. Whereas the earlier Biomed I project was focused on hospital care provided to stroke patients, the follow-up study funded under the Biomed II programme investigated inputs to patient care over a period of 1 year, and therefore included not only the hospital care but also medical care provided in hospital outpatient departments and in primary care settings, as well as social care. Thus a more complex picture of stroke care in different countries was being investigated. We therefore aimed to collect descriptive information about the way in which acute and longer-term stroke care is organised locally and other factors which we assumed might affect care (e.g. expectations about the level of involvement of family members in the care of the elderly), and then to develop a framework for comparing this information across centres.

The problem which we had to consider was how to take into account the effect that different healthcare and social care systems might have on inputs and outcomes. This problem had a number of different aspects, including the following:

- the types of information about healthcare systems which we needed to collect
- how such information could be collected efficiently, and what implications this might have for the adequacy of process indicators being collected

- how we might relate data about the 'structures' of care to the process and outcome data being collected.

By collecting such information we hoped to build up a profile of each centre in order to provide a context in which to set the outcome data being collected, and to collect information which might be helpful when considering explanations for eventual variations in outcome. Since the prospective study was essentially descriptive (patient characteristics, type and quantity of inputs to care, types of outcomes) rather than experimental, the data collected were not random or necessarily 'representative'. Therefore there was no a priori controlling for variables, which made it all the more important to collect information about the specific features of each setting.

Methods of data collection

Audit data-collection questionnaires provided a model for a semi-structured interview schedule which we developed for use in interview with key informants (professionals involved in the delivery of stroke care) in each of the participating centres. The schedule covered a range of issues, including the local healthcare system, characteristics of the admitting hospitals, characteristics of the catchment population, models of care within the hospital, healthcare professionals involved in stroke care, policies with regard to length of stay, discharge planning and destinations, follow-up of patients, provision of services in the community, and roles of family members (*see* Box 4.3).

Box 4.3   Interview topic guide

1   Local healthcare system
2   Hospital (*type, catchment, types of referrals*)
3   Hospital care for stroke patients (*types of ward, admission criteria*)
4   Healthcare professionals providing care for stroke patients
5   Protocols for care/clinical guidelines
6   Hospital policies regarding length of stay
7   Family involvement in inpatient care
8   Planning for discharge (*planning process, discharge destinations*)
9   Follow-up (*providers, organisation*)
10   Rehabilitation (*types of therapy, providers, criteria for access*)
11   Professionals' perceptions of care (*constraints on quality, roles of family*)
12   Routine data collection and other current studies

Interviews were conducted during a site visit to each centre, which also provided an opportunity to discuss data-collection methods, meet other staff involved in data collection, and see at first hand the hospital and other care settings. The site visits were conducted by a team of two or three researchers from the co-ordinating centre, and wherever possible the researchers conducting the visit were from a range of disciplines, including a social scientist, an economist and a clinician. We also asked to interview a range of professionals involved in the delivery of stroke care, including social workers and rehabilitation therapists as well as neurologists and physicians. To allow local professionals to prepare for interviews, a list of topics to be covered was sent prior to the site visit.

All of the visitors took notes during the interview, and on returning to London these were written up by one researcher. Using the interview transcripts, a grid was constructed mapping stroke services across participating centres to allow comparison and identify patterns in service provision. A descriptive report was then written for each centre, which was circulated to the others who had visited the centre and to the relevant study co-ordinator for correction and validation.

Main findings

The findings have been reported elsewhere in greater detail.[21] Below we shall outline the findings for the main areas investigated. Table 4.1 summarises the information collected about the participating centres, and Table 4.2 shows which rehabilitation and community social services were available in the centres at the time of data collection.

Admission routes and inpatient stroke care

In all centres admission to hospital usually occurs following a call to the ambulance service, but local systems have other possible admission routes, including screening by an ambulance physician, primary care doctor or community neurologist. Thus in some centres, the admission of patients may be delayed as they go through local structures, and decisions as to whether and/or where to admit may be outside the control of hospital physicians. This study's approach does not allow an investigation of how stroke patients in different countries recognise the need for help, and of the time intervals to diagnosis and appropriate management in hospital or at home. We were also unable to estimate the variation in admission rates to hospital. Both of these issues could be addressed using the population disease register methodologies described in Chapter 3. Some data relating to delay in admission to hospital are discussed in Chapter 5.

Table 4.1 Participating centres

Centre	Hospital type	Local catchment (population served)	Wards to which stroke patients were admitted
A UK	Teaching	Urban (260 000); significant levels of deprivation and ethnic mix	MDT stroke unit, general medical and elderly care
B France	Teaching/regional specialist centre	Urban (146 000)	MDT stroke unit and neurology
C Germany	Teaching/regional specialist centre	Urban (100 300)	Neurology and dedicated stroke beds
D Germany	Teaching/regional specialist centre	Urban (340 000)	Neurology and acute stroke unit
E Austria	District neurology	Urban (one of 10 units serving 1 600 000)	Neurology
F Denmark	Teaching	Urban (200 000); significant levels of deprivation	MDT stroke unit, neurology and general medical
G Finland	(i) District and (ii) teaching	Urban (165 000)	(i) General medical and (ii) neurology
H Italy	District general	Urban (200 000)	General medical
I Portugal	District general	Urban (350 000); significant levels of deprivation and ethnic mix	Neurology and general medical
J Spain	District general	Urban and rural (67 000)	General medical
K Poland	Teaching	Urban (160 000)	Neurology and dedicated stroke beds
L Lithuania	Teaching/national specialist centre	Urban (420 000)	Neurology
M Latvia	Teaching/national specialist centre	Urban (1 000 000)	Neurology
N Hungary	Teaching/national specialist centre	Urban (200 000)	Neurology and dedicated stroke beds
O Russia	District neurology	Urban (unavailable: 60-bed unit serving two city districts)	Neurology

MDT, multidisciplinary team.

Table 4.2 Rehabilitation and community social services in participating centres

Centre	Rehabilitation pattern	Therapies available	Type of social services available	Patient contribution/means test for home help	Services offered by voluntary sector organisations [a]
Hospital A	IPR and CR	PT, ST and OT	HH, MOW, RC and DC	Yes	Patient groups, home services amd transport
Hospital B	IPR, RU and IPR	PT, ST and CT	HH	Yes	Nil
Hospital C	IPR, RH, OP and P	PT, ST and OT	HH, MOW, RC and DC	Yes[b]	Organise patient groups
Hospital D	IPR, RH, OP and P	PT, ST and OT	HH, MOW, RC and DC	Yes[b]	Organise patient groups
Hospital E	IPR, OP and P	PT, ST and OT	HH, MOW, RC and DC	Yes[b]	Nil
Hospital F	IPR and RH	PT, ST and OT	HH, MOW, RC and DC	No	Organise patient groups
Hospital G	IPR, P and CR	PT, ST and OT	HH, MOW, RC and DC	Yes	Organise patient groups and home services
Hospital H	IPR, RH and CR	PT and ST	HH	Yes	Visits to patients and transport
Hospital I	IPR and OP	PT and ST	HH and MOW	Yes	Home services
Hospital J	IPR, RH and OP	PT	HH and MOW	Yes	Home services and visits to patients
Hospital K	IPR and RH[c]	PT and ST	HH	Yes	Nil
Hospital L	IPR and RH[d]	PT and ST	Nil	Nil	Nil
Hospital M	IPR and RH[e]	PT and ST	Nil	Nil	Nil
Hospital N	IPR and RH	PT and ST	HH	Yes	Nil
Hospital O	IPR	PT	Nil	Nil	Nil

IPR, in-patient rehabilitation; CR, community rehabilitation; RH, rehabilitation hospital; OP, hospital-based outpatient rehabilitation; RU, hospital-based rehabilitation unit; P, privately purchased rehabilitation; PT, physiotherapy; ST, speech therapy; OT, occupational therapy; HH, home help; MOW, meals-on-wheels; RC, respite care; DC, day centre.
[a] Excludes voluntary-sector groups operating as one of a number of providers of social services.
[b] Social insurance system can fund access to services.
[c] Six-month waiting-list; patient must be walking.
[d] Patient must be functionally independent.
[e] Only patients aged <65 years and without comorbidities.

In almost all of the centres stroke patients are cared for by neurologists. General physicians routinely care for stroke patients in the UK centre and the Spanish centre. In both of these countries this reflects the limited neurology services that are available locally. Across the centres stroke patients could be admitted to a range of wards, including stroke units, neurology wards, medical wards or geriatric wards. However, the stroke units are not identical, in some cases having multidisciplinary staff, while another is an acute care unit focusing on intensive monitoring. Still other centres have dedicated stroke beds within neurology wards.

The staffing levels vary widely from one centre to another, reflecting differences in the type of hospital (teaching or non-teaching) and in local levels of trained nurses and doctors in the work-force. To illustrate the range of variation, we calculated the ratio of nurses (excluding nurse auxiliaries) to patients per morning shift. This ranged from $1:3$ to $1:15$. The ratio of qualified doctors (i.e. neurologists or physicians working full-time with stroke inpatients, but excluding neurosurgeons and other consulting specialists) to patients ranged from $1:10$ to $1:18$ in the non-teaching hospitals, and from $1:4.5$ to $1:8.6$ in the teaching hospitals.

An important difference in the trajectory of care concerns the way in which longer-term rehabilitation is provided. In some centres it is routine for patients to be discharged to a separate rehabilitation hospital. In centres where the funding system allows this, all patients generally receive such care. In some Eastern European centres patients who are not functionally independent cannot be admitted to the rehabilitation hospital because of the low nursing levels of the latter. In other centres rehabilitation is provided within the acute setting by on-site therapists.

These different practices have implications for recorded lengths of stay. Obviously, where patients are discharged to another hospital for rehabilitation their lengths of stay in that setting will be reduced. Other factors which were reported as affecting length of stay included financial pressures imposed by hospital management to discharge patients, specific funding mechanisms which imposed upper limits for certain categories of patients and pressure on beds arising from the need to admit new patients.

Rehabilitation therapies

The delivery of rehabilitation therapies and the content of those therapies vary considerably across centres. Therapies are provided in the acute hospital, in rehabilitation units within the hospital, in distinct rehabilitation hospitals, in outpatient clinics and in the community. The types of therapy routinely provided also varied, with some centres having physiotherapy, speech therapy and occupational therapy or cognitive therapy routinely available. In some Eastern European centres only physiotherapy is routinely provided. In still other centres only physiotherapy and speech therapy are available. There were also important differences in the amount of rehabilitation provided (with estimates ranging from 30 minutes per day to a maximum of two sessions per day of up to 90 minutes per session), in the time points at which therapy would begin after the acute event, and in the techniques used.

Family roles

Since some studies have shown that the family plays an important part in caring for stroke patients, particularly after discharge from the acute hospital, we decided to investigate the role that family members were expected to play in participating centres. We were restricted to interviewing health professionals, which limited the investigation to their perceptions and expectations. Nevertheless, differences were found in a number of issues. For example, there were differences in family members' involvement in care during the inpatient stay. It was particularly noticeable, for instance, that in centres with low levels of nursing care, family members were more active, and in one centre were even expected to assist with feeding and washing of the patients. There were also differences in the way in which the family participated in preparations for discharge, with formal consultation of family members going on prior to discharge only in some centres. Similarly, only some centres actively encourage carers to become involved with inpatient rehabilitation. Although it was suggested in all centres that the family is generally the most important resource for patients after discharge, there were differences here, too. For example, in Finland it was reported that it is 'normal' for elderly people to be admitted to social institutions, whereas in Mediterranean and Eastern European centres it was reported that stroke patients would only be admitted to an institution if the family was unable to meet its responsibility to care for the patient after discharge.

Community services

Following discharge from hospital, patients in European centres can expect vastly different levels and types of support. Although domiciliary nursing services exist in all centres for the provision of basic nursing care to chronically ill or disabled patients in the home, in three Eastern European centres this was the only source of community support. In a small number of centres, other services available include meals-on-wheels and respite care. In centres where social insurance systems exist, the level of support that can be provided is greater than in centres where services are financed through general taxation.

In most centres, the voluntary sector does not play a significant role in supporting stroke patients in the community. In the Eastern European centres, this sector is virtually non-existent. In other settings, charitable groups, including church organisations, provide additional or optional services to those organised by the statutory sector, sometimes in a contracted relationship with local authorities. Stroke patient support or advocacy groups exist in only a minority of centres.

Conclusions

Background issues

- Interpretation of outcome data from different settings is not straightforward, even when case-mix variations are adjusted for.
- Differences in patient characteristics do not explain important differences in the provision of care or in patient outcomes.
- The structures and processes of care vary from one locality to the next, particularly when making cross-national comparisons. A major question for the Biomed II stroke study was how to take into account the effect that different health and social care systems might have on care and outcomes.

Methods used in the Biomed II stroke study

- A qualitiative approach involved in-depth interviews with care providers including doctors, nurses, physiotherapists, occupational therapists and social workers.
- A standardised open-ended questionnaire was used to investigate local process of care from admission to provision of care following discharge from the acute setting.
- Using the interview transcripts, a grid was constructed mapping stroke services across participating centres to allow comparison and identify patterns in service provision.

This investigation was systematic, but it may have been limited by the superficial nature of the study, which was imposed of necessity because of limited resources. For example, one particular gap was our inability to capture the perspective of patients and carers. Nevertheless, the exercise was worthwhile for a number of reasons.

Although international guidelines on the care of stroke patients have been produced (e.g. the Helsingborg Declaration 1995),[22] it is clear from the enormous variations in structures and process that the organisation of stroke care is idiosyncratic, reflecting local economic and social contexts rather than objectively defined patient needs.

Box 4.4   Biomed findings/implications

- Using the model of audit, standardised questionnaires/interview schedules can be used to collect information about the processes of care as well as social, political, economic and organisational factors which may affect the uptake and provision of care.
- Until international agreements on standardised measures of stroke severity and other case-mix variables are reached and there are clear links made between treatment and outcome, it may be more appropriate to compare services by the process with which care is delivered and not the health outcomes.
- Such information can be used to:
    review the quality of quantitative data indiciators
    interpret quantitative data
    identify further areas that require investigation.

The descriptive data collected provide contextual information to assist in the interpretation of statistical data gathered in the cohort study. Understanding local structures and processes also allows one to consider what recommendations for changes might realistically be made. For example, insistence on multidisciplinary care for stroke patients may not be helpful in centres where there are few qualified professionals in the workforce and they are poorly paid.

This exercise also encourages consideration of the indicators being used in the quantitative study. For example, although quantitative data were collected on rehabilitation therapies received, it emerged that there were differences in the amounts of therapy, types of therapy practised and time points at which therapy would be initiated. Therefore the degree and complexity of variation highlight the need for caution in assuming that studies which control for patient characteristics thereby control for all relevant variables. Similarly, other differences in clinical practice at the acute stage of illness were observed, and more detailed investigation of these differences has been initiated.

There are similar issues relating to the problems of interpreting outcomes for most chronic diseases. This becomes an increasingly relevant issue for politicians and managers running managed care programmes. Systematic assessments of structure, process and outcome are required in order to develop quality indicators of care for all diseases in whatever setting.

References

1   Davenport RJ, Dennis MS and Warlow CP (1996) Effect of correcting outcome data for case mix: an example from stroke medicine. *BMJ*. **312**: 1503–5.

2   Wolfe CD, Tilling K, Beech R and Rudd AG (1999) Variations in case fatality and dependency from stroke in western and central Europe. The European BIOMED Study of Stroke Care Group. *Stroke*. **30**: 350–6.

3   Stroke Unit Triallists Collaboration (1997) Collaborative systematic review of the randomised controlled trials of organised inpatient (stroke unit) care after stroke. *BMJ*. **314**: 1151–9.

4   Signorini DF, Weir NU and Sandercok P (1999) Variations in clinical outcome in the international trial: implications for international randomised controlled trials. *Cerebrovasc Dis*. **9 (supplement 1)**: 18.

5   Wolfe CDA, Taub NA, Woodrow J, Richardson E, Warburton FG and Burney PGJ (1993) Patterns of acute stroke care in three districts of southern England. *J Epidemiol Commun Health*. **47**: 144–8.

6   Drabkowska-Kaczmarek A, Ignaczak A, Drabkowska K and Nowicka-Sieroszewska K (1983) Care of patients with cerebrovascular disorders in the health service area of one of Warsaw's neurological hospital departments. *Neurol Neuchir Pol*. **17**: 445–51 (abstract).

7   Lee AJ, Huber JH and Stason WB (1997) Factors contributing to practice variation in post-stroke rehabilitation. *Health Serv Res*. **32**: 197–221.

8   Irwin P and Rudd A (1998) Case mix and process indicators of oucome in stroke. The Royal College of Physicians minimum data set for stroke. *J R Coll Phys Lond*. **32**: 442–4.

9   Long AF and Fairfield G (1996) Confusion of levels in monitoring outcomes and/or process. *Lancet*. **347**: 1572.

10 Mackenbach JP, Bouvier-Colle MH and Jougla E (1990) 'Avoidable' mortality and health services: a review of aggregate data studies. *J Epidemiol Commun Health*. **44**: 106–11.

11 Treurniet HF, Looman CW, van der Mass PJ and Mackenbach JP (1999) Variations in 'avoidable' mortality: a reflection of variations in incidence? *Int J Epidemiol*. **28**: 225–32.

12 Rudd AG, Irwin P, Rutledge Z *et al*. (1999) The National Sentinel Audit for Stroke: a tool for raising standards of care. *J R Coll Phys Lond*. **33**: 460–4.

13 Clinical Resource and Audit Group, Chest Heart and Stroke Association, Scotland (1999) *Scottish Stroke Services Audit. Report of an audit on the organisation of services for stroke patients 1997–1998*. Royal College of Physicians, Glasgow.

14 Retchin SM, Brown RS, Yeh SC and Moreno L (1997) Outcomes of stroke patients in Medicare fee-for-service and managed care. *JAMA*. **278**: 119–24.

15 Horner RD, Matchar DB, Divine GW and Feussner JR (1995) Relationship between physician specialty and the selection and outcome of ischemic stroke patients. *Health Serv Res*. **30**: 275–87.

16 Aiken LH, Sloane DM, Lake ET, Sochalski J and Weber AL (1999) Organization and outcomes of inpatient AIDS care. *Med Care*. **37**: 760–72.

17 Good M (1995) Cultural studies of biomedicine. *Soc Sci Med*. **41**: 461–73.

18 Mays N and Pope C (1996) Rigour and qualitative research. In: *Qualitative Research in Health Care*. BMJ Publishing Group, London, 10–19.

19 Abel-Smith B, Figueras J, Holland W, McKee M and Mossialos E (1995) *Choices in Health Policy: an agenda for the European Union*. Office for Official Publications of the European Communities, Luxembourg.

20 Hutten JBF and Kerkstra A (1996) *Home Care in Europe*. Arena, Aldershot.

21 McKevitt C, Beech R, Pound P, Rudd AG and Wolfe CDA (2000) Putting stroke outcomes into context: assessment of variations in the processes of care. *Eur J Pub Health*. **10**: 120–26.

22 World Health Organisation Regional Office for Europe, European Stroke Council (1995) Pan-European Consensus Meeting on Stroke Management, Helsingborg. November.

CHAPTER 5

Variations in the processes of care for stroke: implications for quality improvements

Roger Beech, Ruth Dundas, Domenico Inzitari, Klaus Kunze, Ajay Bhalla and Peter Heuschmann

Introduction

Continuing the themes of measurement of the quality of care, this chapter describes how the process of care between countries and centres can be estimated and presented. The following issues will be discussed:

- the drive to improve quality of care and monitor healthcare activity
- a description of the process data that can be collected for a chronic disease such as stroke across centres and countries.

For defined populations, projects such as the European Union Study of Avoidable Deaths[1] and the MONICA studies[2] have exposed major differences in mortality between and within countries for a range of diagnoses and treatments in younger populations. Likewise, major differences have been observed in case fatality rates between populations with acute myocardial infarction and cancer.[3,4]

Hospital outcomes have also been compared using, for example, confidential enquiries, including that into the study of deaths from cardiac surgery in Bristol.[5,6] Variations in mortality have been exposed, findings which have generated support for the introduction of league tables for comparing mortality rates by hospitals (*see* Chapter 6).

In part, variations in mortality between populations and hospitals reflect differences in the incidence of disease, which in turn reflect differences in the presence of risk factors among populations.[7] In addition, variations reflect differences in the case mix of hospital admissions. However, these factors do not fully account for differences in mortality, and other outcomes. For example, previous research revealed significant differences between hospitals in mortality and disability following stroke, findings which were not explained by differences in the case mix of their stroke admissions.[8]

There is now a growing belief that variations in outcomes between settings may also be due to differences in the ways in which care is delivered.[9] For stroke, previous analysis revealed major variations between European hospitals in the care received by their stroke admissions, and these differences were not explained by variations in the case mix of their patients.[10] For myocardial infarction, major variations have been demonstrated between the USA and Eastern Europe in the delivery of cardiac procedures and the use of coronary-care units.[11]

As a result, there is now a strategic and systematic drive both to standardise and to improve the quality of care processes across settings. In the UK this is reflected in initiatives such as the introduction of systems for clinical governance,[12] the promotion of evidence-based medicine through bodies such as the National Institute for Clinical Excellence,[13] and the use of guidelines and National Service Frameworks to support clinical decision making.[14] For stroke care, various guidelines and consensus statements have been developed, such as the Helsingborg Declaration on Stroke Management[15] and the National Guidelines for Stroke by the Intercollegiate Stroke Working Party.[16] Major national audits have also been completed to assess current standards for stroke care in the UK.[17,18] Elsewhere, the Hamburg Stroke Management Project is a further example of an investigation into standards of care in different hospitals.[19]

Box 5.1

This chapter focuses on the management of stroke and exposes the current baseline, in terms of key processes of care, in a sample of hospitals throughout Europe. Any drive to standardise and improve care processes must start from a baseline, awareness of which allows an assessment of both the need for and feasibility of implementing guideline-supported care.

The data used in this analysis have been generated by the European Union Biomed studies of stroke. These studies have developed registers which collect details of patients' baseline characteristics, as well as information about their strokes, the care they received, and the outcomes of that care. The precise details of the data collected, and the methods of data collection, have been fully reported elsewhere[10] and in other chapters of this book (*see* Chapters 2, 4, 6 and 8).

The results presented here update and extend previous analysis of data from the Biomed I study.[10] In particular, the inclusion of the Biomed II data set means that hospitals from Central and Eastern Europe are now included. This is important, as it is here that upward trends in stroke mortality are now being observed – trends in the opposite direction to those in the remainder of Europe.[20] The principles of data collection and collation have been described in Chapter 2.

The sample of hospitals and patients studied

Details of the hospitals and patients included are listed in Table 5.1. The hospitals are all secondary care general or teaching hospitals in or adjacent to major European cities (Almada is a suburb of Lisbon). Although an analysis of case mix is not the focus of this chapter, selected case-mix variables have been presented to provide a fuller description of the types of patients included. A discussion of how to handle the variation in case mix is provided in Chapter 6.

With the exception of Copenhagen, independence was assessed using the Barthel Index (scale 0–20). In Copenhagen, a Rankin assessment of handicap was used. Stroke type was based on a computed tomography (CT) scan diagnosis. The high proportion of cases in Kaunas, Lithuania, where stroke type was unknown, reflects the low proportion of cases receiving a CT scan (*see* Table 5.2).

Processes of care

The results describe key elements and characteristics of stroke care in the different hospitals. The period of care that was covered starts with the onset of stroke and ends with inpatient discharge from the study hospital.

Initial access to care

The results in Table 5.2 compare the hospitals with regard to the time from stroke onset to admission to acute care and from onset to initial CT scan. In 8 of the 11 hospitals, over 70% of stroke cases were admitted within 24 hours of onset, and over 75% in seven. It is difficult to interpret the results for Copenhagen because of the relatively high proportion of cases for which the time from onset to admission was unknown. As indicated in

Table 5.1 Hospitals and patients

Centre	Number of hospital patients	Mean age (years)	Independent pre-stroke (%)	Stroke diagnosis
Almada, Portugal	111	67.8	78.4	Inf 75 (67.6%) Haem 27 (24.3%) Unknown 9 (8.1%)
Copenhagen, Denmark	318	69.7	69.6	Inf 208 (65.4%) Haem 57 (17.9%) Unknown 53 (16.7%)
Dijon, France	138	73.2	60.1	Inf 127 (92.0%) Haem 6 (4.4%) Unknown 5 (3.6%)
Florence, Italy	155	75.3	61.9	Inf 101 (65.2%) Haem 33 (21.3%) Unknown 21 (13.5%)
Hamburg, Germany	141	68.8	83.0	Inf 104 (73.8%) Haem 21 (14.9%) Unknown 16 (11.3%)
London, UK	108	73.5	75.0	Inf 88 (81.5%) Haem 10 (9.3%) Unknown 10 (9.3%)
Vienna, Austria	96	69.7	71.9	Inf 63 (65.6%) Haem 10 (10.4%) Unknown 23 (24.0%)
Budapest, Hungary	148	62.7	85.8	Inf 108 (73.0%) Haem 33 (22.3%) Unknown 7 (4.7%)
Kaunas, Lithuania	237	71.6	89.0	Inf 15 (6.3%) Haem 13 (5.5%) Unknown 209 (88.2%)
Riga, Latvia	310	64.3	90.0	Inf 105 (33.9%) Haem 61 (19.7%) Unknown 144 (46.4%)
Warsaw, Poland	153	71.9	81.1	Inf 122 (79.7%) Haem 13 (8.5%) Unknown 18 (11.8%)
Overall total	1915	69.9	78.6	Inf 1116 (58.3%) Haem 284 (14.8%) Unknown 515 (26.9%)

Inf, infarct; Haem, haemorrhage.

Table 5.2   Access to key services for patients hospitalised with stroke

Centre	Onset to admission n (%)		Onset to first CT scan n (%)	
Almada, Portugal	<6 hours	47 (42.3%)	<12 hours	58 (52.3%)
	6–24 hours	45 (40.5%)	12–24 hours	28 (25.2%)
	1–7 days	17 (15.3%)	1–7 days	22 (19.8%)
	>7 days	1 (0.9%)	>7 days	2 (1.8%)
	Unknown	1 (0.9%)	Time unknown	0 (0.0%)
			Did not have scan	1 (0.9%)
Copenhagen, Denmark	<6 hours	104 (32.7%)	<12 hours	0 (0.0%)
	6–24 hours	55 (17.3%)	12–24 hours	102 (32.1%)
	1–7 days	50 (15.7%)	1–7 days	89 (28.0%)
	>7 days	16 (5.0%)	>7 days	39 (12.3%)
	Unknown	93 (29.2%)	Time unknown	25 (7.8%)
			Did not have scan	63 (19.8%)
Dijon, France	<6 hours	62 (44.9%)	<12 hours	52 (37.7%)
	6–24 hours	51 (37.0%)	12–24 hours	52 (37.7%)
	1–7 days	20 (14.5%)	1–7 days	28 (20.3%)
	>7 days	3 (2.2%)	>7 days	4 (2.9%)
	Unknown	2 (1.4%)	Time unknown	0 (0.0%)
			Did not have scan	2 (1.4%)
Florence, Italy	<6 hours	2 (1.3%)	<12 hours	100 (64.5%)
	6–24 hours	95 (61.3%)	12–24 hours	17 (11.0%)
	1–7 days	38 (24.5%)	1–7 days	25 (16.1%)
	>7 days	19 (12.3%)	>7 days	1 (0.6%)
	Unknown	1 (0.6%)	Time unknown	10 (6.5%)
			Did not have scan	2 (1.3%)
Hamburg, Germany	<6 hours	42 (29.8%)	<12 hours	78 (55.3%)
	6–24 hours	58 (41.1%)	12–24 hours	36 (25.6%)
	1–7 days	18 (12.8%)	1–7 days	13 (9.2%)
	>7 days	8 (5.7%)	>7 days	4 (2.8%)
	Unknown	15 (10.6%)	Time unknown	9 (6.4%)
			Did not have scan	1 (0.7%)
London, UK	<6 hours	50 (46.3%)	<12 hours	0 (0.0%)
	6–24 hours	34 (31.5%)	12–24 hours	22 (20.4%)
	1–7 days	22 (20.4%)	1–7 days	50 (46.3%)
	>7 days	2 (1.8%)	>7 days	15 (13.9%)
	Unknown	0 (0%)	Time unknown	7 (6.5%)
			Did not have scan	14 (12.9%)
Vienna, Austria	<6 hours	54 (56.3%)	<12 hours	60 (62.5%)
	6–24 hours	21 (21.9%)	12–24 hours	10 (10.4%)
	1–7 days	17 (17.7%)	1–7 days	20 (20.8%)
	>7 days	4 (4.2%)	>7 days	4 (4.2%)
	Unknown	0 (0%)	Time unknown	2 (2.1%)
			Did not have scan	0 (0.0%)
Budapest, Hungary	<6 hours	114 (77.0%)	<12 hours	109 (73.7%)
	6–24 hours	23 (15.6%)	12–24 hours	21 (14.2%)
	1–7 days	7 (4.7%)	1–7 days	12 (8.1%)
	>7 days	3 (2.0%)	>7 days	3 (2.0%)
	Unknown	1 (0.7%)	Time unknown	3 (2.0%)
			Did not have scan	0 (0.0%)

Table 5.2 Continued

Centre	Onset to admission n (%)		Onset to first CT Scan n (%)	
Kaunas, Lithuania	<6 hours	116 (48.9%)	<12 hours	11 (4.6%)
	6–24 hours	65 (27.4%)	12–24 hours	4 (1.7%)
	1–7 days	46 (19.4%)	1–7 days	13 (5.5%)
	>7 days	9 (3.8%)	>7 days	9 (3.8%)
	Unknown	1 (0.5%)	Time unknown	0 (0.0%)
			Did not have scan	200 (84.4%)
Riga, Latvia	<6 hours	108 (34.8%)	<12 hours	127 (41.0%)
	6–24 hours	78 (25.2%)	12–24 hours	60 (19.4%)
	1–7 days	79 (25.5%)	1–7 days	68 (21.9%)
	>7 days	39 (12.6%)	>7 days	37 (11.9%)
	Unknown	6 (1.9%)	Time unknown	9 (2.9%)
			Did not have scan	9 (2.9%)
Warsaw, Poland	<6 hours	74 (48.4%)	<12 hours	0 (0.0%)
	6–24 hours	45 (29.4%)	12–24 hours	74 (48.4%)
	1–7 days	16 (10.5%)	1–7 days	41 (26.8%)
	>7 days	17 (11.1%)	>7 days	34 (22.2%)
	Unknown	1 (0.6%)	Time unknown	1 (0.6%)
			Did not have scan	3 (2.0%)
Overall total	<6 hours	773 (40.4%)	<12 hours	595 (31.1%)
	6–24 hours	570 (29.8%)	12–24 hours	426 (22.2%)
	1–7 days	330 (17.2%)	1–7 days	381 (19.9%)
	>7 days	121 (6.3%)	>7 days	152 (7.9%)
	Unknown	121 (6.3%)	Time unknown	66 (3.4%)
			Did not have scan	295 (15.4%)

previous chapters, this hospital-based study cannot estimate the proportion of stroke patients admitted to hospital, and these data only reflect delay times for patients admitted to hospital.

In 6 of the 11 hospitals over 70% of patients had their first CT scan within 24 hours of onset. These hospitals also tended to have a high proportion of patients scanned within 12 hours of onset.

Use of hospital beds

The results presented in Table 5.3 illustrate the types of beds used for the care of patients in the different hospitals. The statistics cover the bed type on admission and following a subsequent transfer, if applicable.

Use of a clinical data area defined as a stroke unit was common in 6 of the 11 hospitals, but largely absent in the other five. Other common bed types used were those provided by the specialties of internal medicine and neurology. In Dijon, Riga and Warsaw, a large proportion of patients were admitted to beds in intensive-care units.

Table 5.3   Types of bed used by stroke patients and transfers

Centre	Bed type on admission n (%)		Overall number transferred to another bed type n (%)	Second bed type if transferred n (%)	
Almada, Portugal	Internal medicine	111 (100%)	27 (24.3%)	Internal medicine	0 (0.0%)
	Neurology	0 (0%)		Neurology	27 (100%)
	Stroke unit	0 (0%)		Stroke unit	0 (0.0%)
	Other	0 (0%)		Other	0 (0.0%)
Copenhagen,	Internal medicine	108 (34.0%)	59 (18.6%)	Internal medicine	11 (18.6%)
Denmark	Neurology	80 (25.1%)		Neurology	6 (10.2%)
	Stroke unit	96 (30.2%)		Stroke unit	11 (18.6%)
	Other	34 (10.7%)		Other	31 (52.6%)
Dijon, France	Internal medicine	4 (2.9%)	75 (54.3%)	Internal medicine	16 (21.3%)
	Neurology	55 (39.9%)		Neurology	57 (76.0%)
	Stroke unit	0 (0%)		Stroke unit	0 (0%)
	Other	79 (57.2%)		Other	2 (2.7%)
Florence, Italy	Internal medicine	62 (40.0%)	32 (20.6%)	Internal medicine	21 (65.6%)
	Neurology	0 (0.0%)		Neurology	0 (0%)
	Stroke unit	85 (54.8%)		Stroke unit	7 (21.9%)
	Other	8 (5.2%)		Other	4 (12.5%)
Hamburg, Germany	Internal medicine	0 (0%)	29 (20.6%)	Internal medicine	6 (20.7%)
	Neurology	87 (61.7%)		Neurology	17 (58.6%)
	Stroke unit	38 (27.0%)		Stroke unit	4 (13.8%)
	Other	16 (11.3%)		Other	2 (6.9%)
London, UK	Internal medicine	41 (38.0%)	40 (37.0%)	Internal medicine	4 (11.1%)
	Neurology	0 (0.0%)		Neurology	0 (0%)
	Stroke unit	13 (12.0%)		Stroke unit	19 (52.8%)
	Other	54 (50.0%)		Other	17 (36.1%)
Vienna, Austria	Internal medicine	16 (16.7%)	40 (41.7%)	Internal medicine	1 (2.5%)
	Neurology	14 (14.5%)		Neurology	11 (27.5%)
	Stroke unit	57 (59.4%)		Stroke unit	22 (55.0%)
	Other	9 (9.4%)		Other	6 (15.0%)
Budapest, Hungary	Internal medicine	37 (25.0%)	66 (44.6%)	Internal medicine	1 (1.5%)
	Neurology	17 (11.5%)		Neurology	2 (3.0%)
	Stroke unit	82 (55.4%)		Stroke unit	56 (84.9%)
	Other	12 (8.1%)		Other	7 (10.6%)
Kaunas, Lithuania	Internal medicine	0 (0.0%)	33 (13.0%)	Internal medicine	1 (3.0%)
	Neurology	204 (86.1%)		Neurology	7 (21.2%)
	Stroke unit	0 (0.0%)		Stroke unit	0 (0%)
	Other	33 (13.9%)		Other	25 (75.8%)
Riga, Latvia	Internal medicine	0 (0.0%)	14 (4.5%)	Internal medicine	0 (0.0%)
	Neurology	202 (65.2%)		Neurology	5 (35.7%)
	Stroke unit	0 (0.0%)		Stroke unit	1 (7.2%)
	Other	108 (34.8%)		Other	8 (57.1%)
Warsaw, Poland	Internal medicine	0 (0.0%)	75 (49.0%)	Internal medicine	0 (0.0%)
	Neurology	0 (0.0%)		Neurology	0 (0.0%)
	Stroke unit	78 (51.0%)		Stroke unit	75 (100%)
	Other	75 (49.0%)		Other	0 (0.0%)
Overall total	Internal medicine	379 (19.8%)	490 (25.6%)	Internal medicine	61 (12.4%)
	Neurology	659 (34.4%)		Neurology	132 (26.9%)
	Stroke unit	449 (23.4%)		Stroke unit	195 (39.8%)
	Other	428 (22.3%)		Other	102 (20.8%)

Table 5.4   Tests and therapeutic interventions

Centre	Number (percentage) having:					
	Angiography	Echocardio-graphy	Carotid Doppler	Neurosurgery	Carotid surgery	Other vascular surgery
Almada	2 (1.8%)	23 (20.7%)	32 (28.8%)	0 (0.0%)	0 (0.0%)	0 (0.0%)
Copenhagen	0 (0.0%)	101 (31.8%)	105 (33.0%)	16 (5.0%)	0 (0.0%)	0 (0.0%)
Dijon	21 (15.2%)	55 (39.9%)	92 (66.7%)	2 (1.4%)	5 (3.6%)	3 (2.2%)
Florence	12 (7.7%)	67 (43.2%)	75 (48.4%)	1 (0.6%)	3 (1.9%)	1 (0.6%)
Hamburg	27 (19.1%)	78 (55.3%)	118 (83.7%)	4 (2.8%)	1 (0.7%)	1 (0.7%)
London	2 (1.9%)	54 (50.5%)	12 (11.1%)	1 (0.9%)	1 (1.0%)	0 (0.0%)
Vienna	11 (11.5%)	24 (25.0%)	93 (96.9%)	0 (0.0%)	5 (5.2%)	1 (1.0%)
Budapest	18 (12.2%)	143 (96.6%)	147 (99.3%)	6 (4.1%)	12 (8.1%)	3 (2.0%)
Kaunas	11 (4.6%)	10 (4.2%)	11 (4.6%)	10 (4.2%)	0 (0.0%)	0 (0.0%)
Riga	53 (17.1%)	20 (6.4%)	94 (30.3%)	6 (1.9%)	3 (1.0%)	5 (1.6%)
Warsaw	0 (0.0%)	107 (69.9%)	147 (96.1%)	0 (0.0%)	0 (0.0%)	0 (0.0%)
Overall	157 (8.2%)	682 (35.6%)	926 (48.4%)	46 (2.4%)	30 (1.6%)	14 (0.7%)

Use of diagnostic and therapeutic interventions

Results relating to patients' use of tests and interventions are shown in Table 5.4. The percentages of patients who had a CT scan were shown in Table 5.2.

With the exception of Kaunas, where only 15.6% of patients were scanned, a high proportion of patients underwent a CT scan as part of their care. There were wide variations in the percentages of patients who had echocardiography (from 4.2% to 96.6%) and carotid Doppler (from 4.6% to 99.3%). The rate of use of angiography and surgical interventions as part of stroke care was generally low.

Discharge from initial hospital of admission

The results presented in Table 5.5 give stroke patients' average length of stay in the different hospitals and, for those patients who were alive at discharge, their level of independence at discharge (measured by the Barthel Index) and their discharge destination. Although independence at discharge is not a process measure in itself, it does provide a crude indication of the point at which patients are considered to be eligible to move to care processes beyond the inpatient setting. Discharge destination helps to illustrate any differences between settings in the various options available for follow-up care.

There are large differences between hospitals in the average lengths of stay of stroke patients, ranging from 9.8 days to 34.8 days for mean stay and

Table 5.5   Discharge status/destination of stroke patients

Centre	Mean (median) length of stay	Mean (median) Barthel score at discharge	Discharge destination n (%)	
Almada, Portugal	12.0 (9)	11.9 (13)	'Home'	79 (96.3%)
			Other hospital	2 (2.5%)
			Rehabilitation unit	0 (0.0%)
			Other institution	0 (0.0%)
			Unknown	1 (1.2%)
Copenhagen, Denmark	21.9 (14)	16.3 (19)	'Home'	151 (56.3%)
			Other hospital	25 (9.3%)
			Rehabilitation unit	72 (26.9%)
			Other institution	19 (7.1%)
			Unknown	1 (0.3%)
Dijon, France	11.5 (9)	12.8 (14)	'Home'	58 (50.0%)
			Other hospital	4 (3.5%)
			Rehabilitation unit	39 (33.6%)
			Other institution	15 (12.9%)
			Unknown	0 (0.0%)
Florence, Italy	9.8 (8)	11.8 (13)	'Home'	86 (67.7%)
			Other hospital	2 (1.6%)
			Rehabilitation unit	28 (22.0%)
			Other institution	11 (8.7%)
			Unknown	0 (0.0%)
Hamburg, Germany	13.9 (12)	12.9 (14.5)	'Home'	36 (27.5%)
			Other hospital	18 (13.7%)
			Rehabilitation unit	70 (53.4%)
			Other institution	1 (0.8%)
			Unknown	6 (4.6%)
London, UK	34.8 (19)	14.5 (18)	'Home'	61 (81.3%)
			Other hospital	0 (0.0%)
			Rehabilitation unit	0 (0.0%)
			Other institution	10 (13.5%)
			Unknown	3 (4.6%)
Vienna, Austria	34.7 (25)	16.0 (20)	'Home'	65 (73.9%)
			Other hospital	5 (5.7%)
			Rehabilitation unit	10 (11.3%)
			Other institution	8 (9.1%)
			Unknown	0 (0.0%)
Budapest, Hungary	26.6 (22)	14.4 (17)	'Home'	65 (52.8%)
			Other hospital	23 (18.7%)
			Rehabilitation unit	30 (24.4%)
			Other institution	5 (4.1%)
			Unknown	0 (0.0%)
Kaunas, Lithuania	18.1 (17)	15.0 (17)	'Home'	128 (64.3%)
			Other hospital	8 (4.0%)
			Rehabilitation unit	55 (27.6%)
			Other institution	6 (3.0%)
			Unknown	2 (1.0%)

Table 5.5   Continued

Centre	Mean (median) length of stay	Mean (median) Barthel score at discharge	Discharge destination n (%)	
Riga, Latvia	13.5 (13)	16.0 (20)	'Home'	172 (83.5%)
			Other hospital	8 (3.9%)
			Rehabilitation unit	9 (4.4%)
			Other institution	17 (8.2%)
			Unknown	0 (0.0%)
Warsaw, Poland	22.4 (18)	14.7 (17)	'Home'	111 (90.2%)
			Other hospital	7 (5.7%)
			Rehabilitation unit	1 (0.8%)
			Other institution	4 (3.3%)
			Unknown	0 (0.0%)
Overall total	18.9 (14)	14.4 (17)	'Home'	947 (64.3%)
			Other hospital	102 (6.9%)
			Rehabilitation unit	314 (21.3%)
			Other institution	96 (6.5%)
			Unknown	13 (1.0%)

from 8 to 25 days for median stay. There are also variations between hospitals in the average Barthel scores of patients at discharge, ranging from 11.8 to 16.3 for the mean score, and from 13 to 20 for the median score. Finally, the options available, in terms of destination following discharge, vary between hospitals. In Almada, London, Riga and Warsaw it appears that, to a large extent, the patient's home is the only option as a discharge destination. The remaining study hospitals have access to a rehabilitation unit, another hospital and/or another institution for ongoing care.

Discussion of findings

These results demonstrate that it is feasible to generate data which describe variations in the processes of care for stroke in hospitals in different countries. The next stage of the analysis would be an assessment of the extent to which variations in care processes were explained by differences in the case mix of stroke admissions to hospitals, using the types of methods described previously.[10] This information would make it possible to highlight aspects of care where a change in practice might be justified in order to improve the quality of care. A change would be indicated if current care processes differed from those suggested by guidelines, consensus statements or other scientific evidence.

Such use of the information that is generated is illustrated below by a discussion of the issues of quality of care that are raised by the analysis presented in this chapter. For the purposes of this discussion it is assumed that the key differences and similarities in the care processes of the hospitals included would have remained after any adjustment for case mix. Such a working assumption is consistent with the results of a previous analysis which demonstrated that adjustment for case mix explains some but not all of the differences in care processes between settings.[10]

Initial access to care

The approach taken in this study limits access issues to individuals hospitalised with stroke. In 8 of the 11 hospitals, over 70% of patients were admitted within 24 hours of stroke onset, and in all of them the figure was over 50%. It is important for some patients to gain access to hospital services as soon as possible in order to undergo urgent evaluation and confirmation of stroke diagnosis. If acute therapies such as thrombolysis are to be introduced, it will be crucial for patients to present within the narrow therapeutic time window of 3 to 6 hours if they are to be eligible for such treatment.[21] The results presented here indicate that there are still considerable delays with regard to hospital admission.

There was considerable variation between the hospitals in the time to first CT scan. In five hospitals over 50% of patients were scanned within 12 hours of admission, whereas in other hospitals most initial scans took place between 12 hours and 7 days after stroke onset. Over 20% of patients in the Warsaw centre were scanned 1 week after stroke onset, and in the centres in London, Copenhagen and Kaunas, 12%, 19% and 84% of patients, respectively, were not scanned.

There is currently uncertainty about the link between brain imaging and stroke outcome, although if thrombolysis is to be offered to subgroups of stroke patients, scanning within a few hours of stroke will be necessary. There are no evidence-based guidelines indicating the correct time for undergoing brain imaging, although guidelines derived from expert opinions or consensus working groups indicate that the majority of scans should be undertaken within 48 hours of stroke onset. If these guidelines are accepted, the results presented here indicate that in this sample of hospitals there is still a need to improve the speed of access to scanning, not only for diagnosis but also for secondary prevention.

Use of hospital beds

Across centres, stroke care is managed by different specialists, namely stroke physicians, neurologists, geriatricians and general physicians. However, it has been argued that emergency evaluation by neurologists enhances the diagnostic accuracy with regard to stroke patients.[22] In the UK there are relatively few neurologists, but there is still controversy as to whether a neurologist rather than an internal physician or geriatrician should manage all stroke patients.[23] In a recent survey in the UK, only 3% of consultants managing stroke patients were specialists in stroke medicine.[18]

A high proportion of the patients treated in Dijon, Riga and Warsaw were initially managed in intensive-care units, reflecting an aggressive approach to critical-care management. However, the question of whether or not this type of care is beneficial in improving stroke outcome remains unanswered.

A finding that initially seems surprising is the low rate of use of stroke units. These were largely absent in 5 of the 11 hospitals, despite the fact that care in a stroke unit had been shown to be the single most important development in stroke care for many years.[24] However, these results must be viewed with caution.

There is no single definition of a stroke unit. Some have a rehabilitation-driven focus, while others have a combined acute and rehabilitation focus. As well as the elements of care provided, differences also include the time of admission to such units.[25] Site visits for the Biomed study confirmed that the label 'stroke unit' is currently attached to settings ranging from a low-technology rehabilitation unit to a highly intensive acute unit. Thus without a uniform definition of the constituents of a stroke unit it is difficult to reach conclusions about the need for a change in care processes in different settings.

Use of diagnostic and therapeutic interventions

With the exception of the centres in Kaunas, the vast majority of patients who were admitted to the study hospitals had a CT scan as part of their care. It is unclear at present whether or not CT scanning actually influences mortality and morbidity. However, the Helsingborg declaration states that all stroke patients admitted to a hospital should have a CT scan to determine the stroke diagnosis and the cause of stroke.[15]

Other therapeutic interventions, such as the use of echocardiography and carotid Doppler, varied in uptake across centres. Echocardiography is often used in an attempt to identify cardio-embolic causes of stroke, although evidence of its effectiveness for this purpose is only available from consensus statements. The use of carotid Doppler should only be considered for patients who would appear to benefit from carotid surgery (i.e. patients with carotid artery area stroke and minor residual ability).[26] The results presented here indicate that if a link does currently exist between rates of carotid Doppler and surgery, it is only minor.

Discharge from initial hospital of admission

There was considerable variation between centres with regard to length of stay, discharge Barthel score and discharge destination. The findings with regard to length of stay confirm those of previous analyses of Biomed data.[10]

The extent to which these variations represent differences in the quality of care is unclear. However, the scale of the variation does indicate a need for more research into the link between stroke outcomes and variations in the overall organisation and processes of care. Such research will help to identify which patterns of care are most clinically effective and cost-effective.

Conclusion

The introduction to this chapter demonstrated that there is now a strategic and systematic drive both to standardise and to improve the quality of care processes for all diseases across settings. Drives to improve the quality of healthcare must start from an understanding of the current baseline in terms of care processes. Projects such as the Biomed studies of stroke, and the methods that they have developed, allow this baseline to be exposed. The study of stroke has enabled many of the issues relating to all diseases to be teased out, as stroke has both an acute and a longer-term healthcare impact.

A knowledge of the baseline of care processes has implications for both the relevance and feasibility of efforts to disseminate guidelines and evidence-based care. Clarification of the baseline, and how it relates to 'good' practice, may also act as a springboard for developments which aim to improve the quality of healthcare. This has happened in the UK, where concern about the existing quality of care has resulted in the establishment of bodies such as the National Institute for Clinical Excellence[13] and the Commission for Health Improvement.[12]

This chapter has focused on hospital care for the treatment of stroke. Its main conclusions can be summarised as follows:

- It is possible to make cross-national comparisons of care processes within hospitals.
- The results of such comparisons help to highlight aspects of care where a change in the delivery of services might be justified in order to improve the quality of care.
- However, the ease with which the information that is generated can be used to make firm policy recommendations about changes in care processes within individual hospitals is affected by the ability to adjust adequately for differences in the case mix of hospitals, by differences

between hospitals in the ways in which individual elements of care are defined (e.g. in the definition of a stroke unit), and by the current lack of evidence about the effectiveness and cost-effectiveness of many elements of care and hence the lack of evidence as to whether or not a change in practice is desirable.

- Therefore the results of such an analysis support, but do not prescribe, decisions about changes in care processes. For some interventions in stroke care, there is evidence that the process of care has an impact on outcome. For other interventions this link is not as well established and needs to be more clearly demonstrated before major recommendations can be made about redesigning services.

References

1 Holland WW (1991) *European Community Atlas of Avoidable Death.* Oxford University Press, Oxford.

2 WHO MONICA Project Principal Investigators (prepared by H Tunstall-Pedoe) (1988) The World Health Organisation MONICA project (monitoring of trends and determinants in cardiovascular diseases): a major international collaboration. *J Clin Epidemiol.* **41**: 105–14.

3 Tunstall-Pedoe H, Kuulasmaa K, Amouyel P, Arveeiler D, Rajakangas A and Pajak A (1994) Myocardial infarction and coronary deaths in the World Health Organisation. MONICA project. *Circulation.* **90**: 583–612.

4 Sikora K (1999) Cancer survival in Britain. *BMJ.* **319**: 461–2.

5 English TAH, Bailey AR, Dark JF and Williams WG (1984) The UK cardiac surgical register 1977–82. *BMJ.* **289**: 1205–8.

6 Treasure T, Taylor K and Black N (1997) *Independent Review of Adult Cardiac Surgery.* United Bristol Health Care Trust, Bristol.

7 Wolfe CDA, Taub NA, Woodrow J, Richardson E, Warburton FG and Burney PGJ (1993) Patterns of acute stroke care in three districts of southern England. *J Epidemiol Community Health.* **47**: 144–8.

8 Wolfe CDA, Tilling K, Beech R and Rudd AG (1999) Variations in case fatality and dependency from stroke in Western and Central Europe. *Stroke.* **30**: 350–6.

9 Treasure T (1998) Lessons from the Bristol case: more openness on risks and on individual surgeons' performance. *BMJ.* **316**: 1685–6.

10 Beech R, Ratcliffe M, Tilling K and Wolfe CDA (1996) Hospital services for stroke care: a European perspective. *Stroke.* **27**: 1958–64.

11 Rosamund W, Broda G, Kawalec E *et al.* (1999) Comparison of medical care and survival of hospitalised patients with acute myocardial infarction in Poland and the United States. *Am J Cardiol.* **83**: 1180–85.

12   Department of Health (1998) *A First-Class Service: quality in the new NHS.* Department of Health, London.

13   Smith R (1999) NICE: a panacea for the NHS? *BMJ.* **318**: 823–4.

14   Tyrer P (1999) The National Service Framework: a scaffold for mental health. *BMJ.* **319**: 1017–18.

15   World Health Organisation Regional Office for Europe, European Stroke Council (1995) Pan European Consensus Meeting on Stroke Management, Helsingborg. November.

16   Royal College of Physicians Intercollegiate Working Party for Stroke (2000) National clinical guidelines for stroke. *J R Coll Phys Lond.* **34**: 131–3.

17   Rudd AG, Irwin P, Rutledge Z, Lowe D, Wade DT and Pearson M (1999) The National Sentinel Audit: an old tool for raising standards of care. *J R Coll Phys Lond.* **33**: 460–4.

18   Ebrahim S and Redfern J (1999) *Stroke Care – a matter of chance.* A national survey of stroke services commissioned by the Stroke Association, London.

19   Kunze K, Christiansen W, Berger J, Forster M and Leffmann C (1998) Das Hamburger Schlaganfallprojekt: Ein Qualitatssicherungsprojekt. *Nervenheilkunde.* **17**: S15–20.

20   Bonita R, Stewart A and Beaglehole R (1990) International trends in stroke mortality: 1970–1985. *Stroke.* **21**: 989–92.

21   Bogousslavsky J, Brott T, Diener HC *et al.* (1996) The European Ad Hoc Consensus Group. European strategies for early intervention in stroke: a report of an Ad Hoc Consensus Group Meeting. *Cerebrovasc Dis.* **6**: 315–24.

22   Lyrer A, Ebnoter A, Operscall E, Rickenbacher C and Steck P (1995) *The effect of introducing a comprehensive stroke program on primary diagnostic evaluation in stroke patients.* Pan European Consensus Meeting on Stroke Management, November 1995, Helsingborg, Sweden. World Health Organisation, Geneva.

23   Heron J, Wilkinson I and Warlow C (1994) Should patients with stroke see a neurologist? *Lancet.* **343**: 544.

24   Stroke Unit Trialists' Collaboration (1997) Collaborative systematic review of the randomised trials of organised inpatient (stroke unit) care after stroke. *BMJ.* **314**: 1151–9.

25   Indredavik B, Bakke F, Slordahl SA, Rokseth R and Haheim LL (1999) Treatment in a combined acute and rehabilitation stroke unit. *Stroke.* **30**: 917–23.

26   European Carotid Surgery Trialists' Collaboration Group (1998) Randomised trial of endarterectomy for recently symptomatic carotid stenosis: final results of the MRC European carotid surgery trial (ECST). *Lancet.* **351**: 1379–87.

CHAPTER 6

League tables of outcome for chronic disease

Kate Tilling, Klaus Kunze and Roger Beech

Background issues

Previous chapters have addressed the issues surrounding the collection and comparison of data on the structure and process of care. This chapter begins to explore how outcome can be assessed and compared across centres, using hospital stroke registers as an example.

A league table can be regarded as any set of units (e.g. schools) arranged in order of an outcome (e.g. examination results), showing the ranking of each unit. Such tables can be used to provide information (e.g. on which type of school performs best in examinations) and also to inform choices (e.g. between several local schools).

League tables in health

There are many potential units for a league table in health, including countries, area, health authorities, hospitals, wards or individual clinicians. The potential benefits of such league tables include monitoring and improving the quality of health care (e.g. by comparing similar wards across a health authority and identifying the worst performers), and informing patient, provider and purchaser choice.

Comparison of surgical outcomes has been a topic of interest for many years, with the first case for uniform surgical statistics for comparative purposes being put forward by Florence Nightingale in 1860.[1] She claimed that the introduction of these uniform statistics would enable comparisons to be made between wards, hospitals and different countries. However, there are problems which limit the use of naive comparisons of statistics, such as mortality rates,[2] including the following:

- the possibility of manipulation of the data
- the need for an outcome other than mortality
- the need for adjustment for comorbidities, markers of disease severity and any other confounding factors before making comparisons.

A joint meeting of forums on quality in healthcare and measurement in medicine was held in 1995[3] to discuss league tables for healthcare. Problems for outcome measurement were identified, and some key criteria for useful league tables were identified, including the following:

- outcomes should be objective, clearly defined (e.g. death) and measured at precise time intervals
- it should be possible to measure outcomes precisely, or inter-observer variation may cause problems with comparability
- league tables should inform the management of the service, and lead to a more informed choice for patients.

It was concluded that effective league tables would not be easy or quick to develop, and would not reflect all aspects of the service. However, one speaker felt that publicly available league tables would help to 'quantify and make explicit the product of the service'.[3]

One study has examined the sensitivity of both death rates and measures of process to differences in the quality of care provided in the treatment of patients with myocardial infarction.[4] A systematic review of the literature was used to identify processes of care for which there was strong evidence of an effect on mortality. This information was used to simulate the mortality rate in a hospital that was not using any of the effective interventions, and in one with varying uptake of the effective interventions. These simulations showed that the sample sizes needed to detect differences in mortality would be much higher than those needed to detect the differences in the process of care leading to the effect on mortality. This may imply that, where there is prior evidence which shows that a few interventions are effective, measures of process rather than outcome could be used for audit and league-table purposes. The authors point out that an observed difference in process between two units is easy to modify, whereas to influence mortality one must first identify the causes of the difference in mortality between units.

There is currently increasing use of comparative outcome indicators in healthcare. In England, Wales and Scotland there is public dissemination of hospital-specific outcome measures such as death within 30 days after an operation. Population outcome indicators are calculated at a health authority level and published in the public health common data set, with regions of England ranked for each indicator. Recent controversies, such as the high death rate associated with certain paediatric surgeons at Bristol,[5] have increased interest in publicly available data both to monitor outcomes and to inform choice. However, unless the league tables are of high quality, and correctly presented and analysed, they may lead to misinformation and to poor decisions making.

League tables in stroke

The Scottish Stroke Outcomes Group has examined the use of routinely collected data as informal league tables. Although such data could be used to rank hospitals, they may be of inadequate quality and lack adequate adjustment for case mix. The Scottish Stroke Outcomes Group examined the mortality and functional status data for five hospitals, and compared the crude data with the results when adjusted using externally validated logistic regression models, including case-mix variables. Adjustment for case mix changed the rank order of the five hospitals for both outcomes, and reduced the variation in outcome between the hospitals.[6]

An International Stroke Trial used data on death and functional dependence from 36 countries to examine variation in outcome between countries. There was less variation between countries in death than in dependency, indicating that some of the variation may be due to differences in the definition and assessment of functional dependence between countries. After adjustment for case mix, three countries had significantly worse and four had significantly better 14-day case fatality than the overall average. When the outcome of death or dependency at 6 months was examined, 16 countries had significantly better than average outcome (after adjustment for case mix), compared with one country with worse than average outcome.[7]

Some information on outcome across different centres or countries may be interpreted as league tables, even though this is not the purpose for which the data were collected. One example of this is the presentation of data from the MONICA study, where incidence and outcome data from different countries are shown in order.[8]

The importance of correcting for case mix was emphasised by a comparison of the crude and case-mix-adjusted effect of treatment in a stroke unit on mortality and morbidity.[9] The crude data showed that individuals who were treated by the organised stroke service were more likely to be alive, independent and living at home 12 months post stroke than those treated in the hospital before the service was introduced. Adjustment for case mix showed non-significant effects of the stroke service on each of these outcomes. A response to this paper noted that wide variation in the variables used in adjustment could lead to erroneous conclusions, and that few routine data sets would be able to collect detailed case-mix information.[10]

Current knowledge

Confidence intervals

A league table is often created merely by ordering the units of comparison (hospitals, countries, individual surgeons) by the statistic of interest (mortality rate, incidence of coronary heart disease). Such a table is easy to interpret, and it is obvious which units are at the top and which are at the bottom. However, there is uncertainty in both the outcome and the rank of each unit, which is not shown by a crude league table. For example, a league table of countries ranked in order of their stroke mortality rates would show the same rankings irrespective of the accuracy with which the mortality rates had been estimated. Two adjacently ranked countries could have confidence intervals with a wide degree of overlap, indicating uncertainty about the actual ranking of these countries.

Many ordered tables of outcome do show confidence intervals around the estimate of outcome. For example, a study of league tables for mortality after acute myocardial infarction[11] shows 31 hospitals ordered by the odds of mortality (standardised for individual, hospital and area risk factors such as age, sex, and Carstairs score of area of residence). The confidence intervals around the odds ratios were also shown, and these indicated that there was a high degree of overlap between the hospitals' mortality odds. This is a useful display of the degree of uncertainty about the odds, but does not enable the viewer to determine easily which units are different, or how large the difference between them may be. For example, two units with slightly overlapping confidence intervals may or may not be significantly different (as tested using a hypothesis test), and the confidence interval for the difference cannot be obtained from such a diagram.

If the league tables are to be used to rank units in order of outcome, then confidence intervals around those ranks must also be presented.[12] One example has applied this methodology to a league table of adjusted live birth rates from 52 *in-vitro* fertilisation clinics.[13] A simulation procedure was used to generate confidence intervals around the rank for each unit. The confidence intervals around the ranks were wider than those around the adjusted live birth rates. Those hospitals with ranks in the middle of the table had particularly wide confidence intervals — the clinic ranked 25th had a 95% confidence interval from 15th to 36th from the bottom of the table. As with other confidence interval calculations, confidence intervals for units with small samples tended to be wider than those for units with large samples.

Adjusting for risk

When adjusting for risk between units of comparison, different levels of measurement need to be taken into account. For example, there are individual-level risk factors which the hospital cannot influence (e.g. age, sex, premorbid conditions), hospital-level risk factors (indicator of average case complexity) and also area-level risk factors (e.g. access to health services, socio-economic status). One problem that is encountered when presenting analyses based on adjusted risk is that different centres may perform better for patients with different risk factors. Thus in the study of mortality following acute myocardial infarction, adjusted odds of death were presented both for patients aged 70 years and for patients aged 50 years, as the same units did not perform best for both groups.[11] This is one reason why a league table of outcomes may not necessarily inform choice for an individual patient.

Multi-level models[14] can be used to adjust for risk, taking into account the fact that patients from any given unit are likely to show some similarity in their outcomes compared with patients from a different unit. These models assume that there is some true underlying rate of outcome, and that the outcome rate for each unit is a random variable drawn from the distribution of the true rate. This has the effect that, when using multi-level models to model rates of outcome, 'shrinkage' tends to occur, whereby the estimated rates are all moved closer to the average rate.[12] Multi-level logistic modelling has been used to adjust for individual-, hospital- and area-level risk factors in a study of league tables for mortality associated with acute myocardial infarction.[11]

The importance of adjusting for comorbidities and disease severity was emphasised in a study of variation in outcome after acute gastrointestinal haemorrhage.[15] A total of 74 hospitals were ranked with regard to crude mortality rates, and then for mortality rates adjusted for a risk score derived from known risk factors. The adjusted rates showed less variation than the unadjusted rates, and 21 hospitals had an adjusted rank which differed from the unadjusted rank by at least 10 places. The authors concluded that, using routine data, only basic adjustment for case mix can be made, and thus league tables of mortality could provide an inaccurate picture of the quality of care. A study of league tables of mortality in neonatal care units confirmed the need to adjust for case mix, as again adjusted and unadjusted mortality rates differed, and changed the rank order of the centres.[16]

Biomed findings

As discussed in earlier chapters and elsewhere,[17,18] there were substantial variations in case mix, process and outcome measures at 3 months post stroke between the 12 centres in Biomed I. Two important outcomes which could be used to form a league table of centres are death by 3 months post stroke, and whether the patient was functionally independent (Barthel Index = 20) at 3 months post stroke.

Death by 3 months post stroke

Figure 6.1 shows the probability of death by 3 months for each of the 12 centres, together with the 95% confidence intervals for probability of death. The horizontal line is the mean probability of death by 3 months for the entire data set (0.31). According to this graph, only the bottom four centres (UK5, UK4, UK3 and UK2) and the best three centres (FR, GE1 and HU) have outcomes that are significantly different from the average probability of death. It can also be seen that although the centres are ordered from lowest to highest probability of death, ranking them would not be a simple matter, as so many of the confidence intervals overlap.

An adjusted probability of death was calculated using a random effects logistic model with death as the outcome, and allowing for correlations between and within centres. Although standardised data collection had taken place, there were few risk factors which were felt to be robust in their

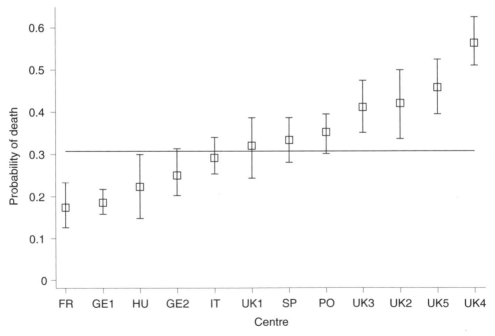

Figure 6.1 Probability of death by 3 months for each centre, with 95% confidence intervals.

interpretation and which had been collected for a large proportion of the data set which could be included in the model. Demographic factors included age, sex and pre-stroke Rankin score. Stroke-severity factors (measured at the time of maximum impairment) included incontinence, loss of consciousness and presence of limb weakness or paralysis. There were significant differences between the centres in all of these variables.[17]

The 95% confidence intervals for the adjusted probabilities were calculated using bootstrap methods as follows. A total of 100 random samples of the data set were taken, and the multi-level logistic model was fitted to each data set and used to calculate the probability of death for the whole initial data set as if they had been treated in each centre. These 100 values can then be regarded as typical of the distribution of the probability, so the 95% confidence interval can be calculated by using the 2.5th and 97.5th centile values. All analyses were performed using Stata software, with an extension to the bootstrap to take into account any bias in the estimates.[19]

Figure 6.2 shows the adjusted probability of death for each centre (averaged over the entire initial data set). The order of the centres has changed from the unadjusted order (*see* Figure 6.1), and there is still a great deal of overlap between the confidence intervals. The adjusted confidence intervals tend to be wider than the unadjusted confidence intervals, so any ordering

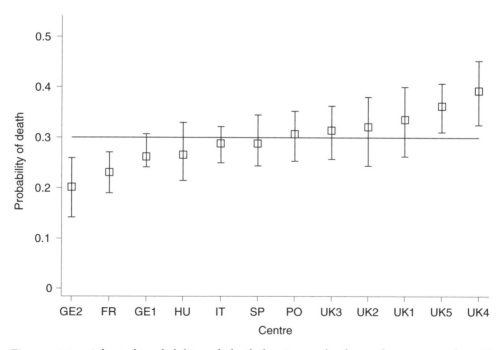

Figure 6.2   Adjusted probability of death by 3 months for each centre, with 95% confidence intervals.

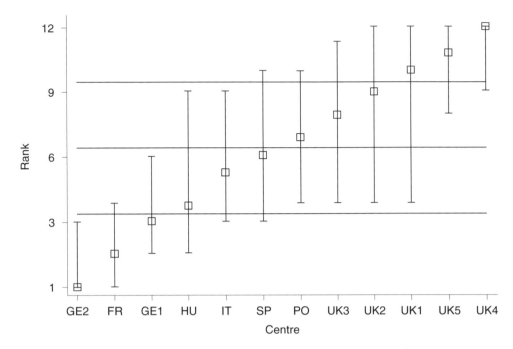

Figure 6.3   Adjusted rank of probability of death by 3 months for each centre, with 95% confidence intervals.

of the centres based on this figure alone would be subject to a great deal of uncertainty. This uncertainty is illustrated in Figure 6.3, where the centres are shown in order of their ranks for death as an outcome (with a rank of 1 being the best centre for this outcome), and with 95% confidence intervals around the ranks. One of the few firm conclusions to be drawn from this graph is that the second German centre and the French centre are likely to be among the top three and four centres, respectively, whilst the fifth and fourth UK centres are likely to be among the bottom five and four centres, respectively. The first German centre is likely to be in the top half of the table. However, all of the confidence intervals for the ranks of the other centres are too wide to provide any useful information.

Independence in activities of daily living (ADL) by 3 months post stroke

Figure 6.4 shows the probability of a poor outcome (death or a Barthel score of < 20) at 3 months for each of the 12 centres, together with the 95% confidence intervals for probability of a poor outcome. The horizontal

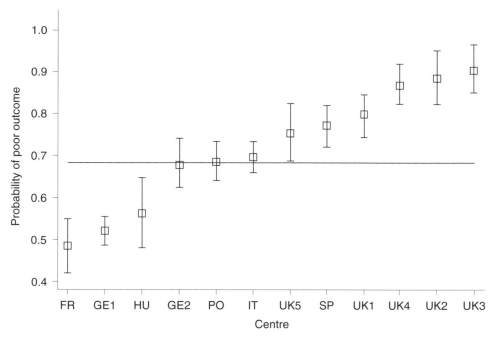

Figure 6.4 Probability of poor outcome by 3 months for each centre, with 95% confidence intervals.

line is the mean probability of a poor outcome by 3 months for the entire data set (0.68). There is more variation in the crude probability of poor outcome than there was in the crude probability of death. The bottom six centres (SP and the five UK centres) all have higher than average probabilities of poor outcome, and the top three centres (FR, GE1 and HU) have lower than average probabilities of poor outcome.

As with probability of death, the probability of poor outcome was adjusted for age, sex, pre-stroke Rankin score, incontinence, loss of consciousness and limb weakness or paralysis. The adjusted probabilities of poor outcome for the initial data set were calculated for each centre, together with 95% confidence intervals (again using bootstrap methods). Figure 6.5 shows the adjusted probabilities of poor outcome, again showing a difference in ranking between adjusted and unadjusted probabilities. The uncertainty with regard to the ordering of the centres with respect to poor outcome is shown in Figure 6.6. As with the ranks for probability of death, the confidence intervals around the ranks are much wider than those around the predicted probabilities. Figure 6.6 shows that the French centre is likely to be ranked highest or second-highest with regard to having a good outcome, and the first, second and third UK centres are likely to be in the bottom four centres. The two German centres and the centre in Hungary are likely to be among

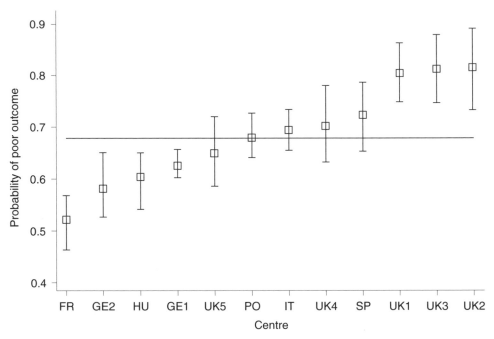

Figure 6.5 Adjusted probability of poor outcome by 3 months for each centre, with 95% confidence intervals.

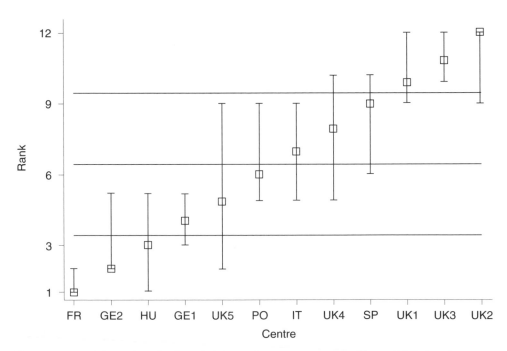

Figure 6.6 Adjusted rank of probability of poor outcome by 3 months for each centre, with 95% confidence intervals.

the top five centres, and the centres in Portugal, Italy and Spain and the fourth UK centre are likely to be ranked somewhere between fifth and tenth. The fifth UK centre has the widest confidence interval, with its true rank likely to be between second and ninth.

Conclusions

* Unadjusted comparisons of outcome between centres can be very misleading.
* Adjustment of outcomes for confounding factors such as case mix and socio-economic status is not straightforward.
* League tables of outcome for subgroups of patients may be an alternative to multiple adjustment, but large samples would be required.
* Measurement of outcome in a standardised fashion to a fixed time point, rather than to discharge from hospital, will reduce the bias in interpretation.
* Further in-depth studies of the reasons behind the variation in outcome are required if quality is to be improved.

One obvious implication of the work presented here is that comparisons of units on unadjusted outcomes can be very misleading. However, adjustment is not straightforward. Even with a standardised data set such as the one used here, there is a limit to the number of useful risk factors which can be collected with sufficient accuracy and cross-centre consistency to be useful. When using routine data sets, the selection of adjustment factors could be a major problem. The order of the centres here relating to stroke was different when comparing adjusted with unadjusted outcomes. It must therefore be borne in mind that had more detailed case-mix and demographic variables been available to use in adjustment, the order of the centres might well have changed.

One particularly useful case-mix adjustment would be adjustment for socio-economic status. However, there are problems with the definition of socio-economic status for older people – the age-group most likely to be affected by stroke – because the definition is based on occupation. It is possible that currently unmeasurable differences in socio-economic class between the patients in the different countries could account for some of the variation in outcome.

Another aspect of adjustment is that there was evidence of interactions between centre and risk factors for both outcomes. For death, there was a significant interaction between centre and incontinence, such that the order of outcome for individuals with and without incontinence was quite different. For independence in ADL, an interaction was apparent between centre and limb paralysis or weakness, again with the order of centres being different for those with and without limb deficit. If league tables such as these were to be used to inform patient or purchaser choice, this difference in outcome would affect the decisions made. Presenting league tables for subgroups of patients is one solution, but it is only practicable with sufficiently large sample sizes. Instead, these differences might inform further investigation into how management at the different centres might vary with these patient characteristics.

League tables should only be drawn up to compare outcomes which have been consistently collected and which have the same meanings across all of the units being compared. Mortality is a suitable outcome for comparison, provided that death is ascertained with the same accuracy in all centres. In this study only stroke patients who were admitted to hospital were used, and there may be a systematic bias in the proportion of patients who died at home or in accident and emergency departments in the different settings. When adjusting for risk factors, we used the entire initial data set to create the comparisons, and thus the estimates should be unbiased provided that the model used fits both the observed and the missing data. There may be some inconsistency in the measurement and interpretation of the Barthel Index between centres or between countries. However, the general pattern of ranking is the same for both outcomes, indicating that this outcome is fairly robust.

There is no point in drawing up league tables and identifying the best and worst units unless the reasons behind these variations are to be sought. It may be that ongoing, in-depth research into the process of care within these 12 centres, and the family and social networks supporting the patients in these areas, might provide an insight into the apparent differences in outcome shown here. On the basis of a (non-random) sample of 12 centres it will be difficult to draw any firm conclusions. However, factors may emerge which could be tested as hypotheses in future prospective studies, and could thus help to raise the standard of stroke care throughout Europe.

References

1   Spiegelhalter DJ (1999) Surgical audit: statistical lessons from Nightingale and Codman. *J R Stat Soc Series A.* **162**: 45–58.
2   Schneider EC and Epstein AM (1996) Influence of cardiac-surgery performance reports on referral practices and access to care. A survey of cardiovascular specialists. *NEJM.* **335**: 251–6.
3   Shaw CD and Costain DW (1995) League tables for health-care. *J R Soc Med.* **88**: 54–7.

4 Mant J and Hicks N (1995) Detecting differences in quality of care: the sensitivity of measures of process and outcome in treating acute myocardial infarction. *BMJ.* **311**: 793–6.

5 Treasure T (1998) Lessons from the Bristol case. More openness – on risks and on individual surgeons' performance. *BMJ.* **316**: 1685–6.

6 Weir N, on behalf of the Scottish Stroke Outcomes Group (1999) Stroke league tables: are they likely to reflect differences in quality? *Cerebrovasc Dis.* **9**: 115.

7 Signorini DF, Weir NU and Sandercock PAG, for the First Collaborative Group (1999) Variations in clinical outcome by country in the International Stroke Trial: implications for international randomised controlled trials. *Cerebrovasc Dis.* **9** (**Supplement 1**): 36.

8 Thorvaldsen P, Asplund K, Kuulasmaa K, Rajakangas AM and Schroll M (1995) Stroke incidence, case fatality and mortality in the WHO MONICA project. World Health Organization monitoring trends and determinants in cardiovascular disease. *Stroke.* **26**: 361–7.

9 Davenport RJ, Dennis MS and Warlow CP (1996) Effect of correcting outcome data for case mix: an example from stroke medicine. *BMJ.* **312**: 1503–5.

10 Barer D, Ellul J and Watkins C (1996) Correcting outcome data for case mix in stroke medicine. Structure and process should be audited, rather than outcomes. *BMJ.* **313**: 1005–6.

11 Leyland AH and Boddy FA (1998) League tables and acute myocardial infarction. *Lancet.* **351**: 555–8.

12 Goldstein H and Spiegelhalter DJ (1996) League tables and their limitations: statistical issues in comparisons of institutional performance. *J R Stat Soc Series A.* **159**: 385–409.

13 Marshall EC and Spiegelhalter DJ (1998) Reliability of league tables of *in-vitro* fertilisation clinics: retrospective analysis of live birth rates. *BMJ/* **316**: 1701–4.

14 Goldstein H (1995) *Multilevel Statistical Models* (2e). Edward Arnold, London.

15 Rockall TA, Logan RF, Devlin HB and Northfield TC (1995) Variation in outcome after acute upper gastrointestinal haemorrhage. The National Audit of Acute Upper Gastrointestinal Haemorrhage. *Lancet.* **346**: 346–50.

16 Parry GJ, Gould CR, McCabe CJ and Tarnow-Mordi WO (1998) Annual league tables of mortality in neonatal intensive-care units: longitudinal study. International Neonatal Network and the Scottish Neonatal Consultants and Nurses Collaborative Study Group. *BMJ.* **316**: 1931–5.

17 Wolfe CDA, Tilling K, Beech R and Rudd AG (1999) Variations in case fatality and dependency from stroke in Western and Central Europe. *Stroke.* **30**: 350–56.

18   Beech R, Ratcliffe M, Tilling K and Wolfe C (1996) Hospital services for stroke care. A European perspective. European Study of Stroke Care. *Stroke.* **27**: 1958–64.

19   Stata Corporation (1997) *Stata Statistical Software: release 5.0.* Stata Corporation, College Station, TX.

CHAPTER 7

From the patient's perspective: subjective outcome assessment

*Christopher McKevitt, Ruth Dundas
and India Remedios*

Subjective outcomes in the context of outcome assessment

This chapter will review the potential place of subjective outcomes in the assessment of outcome, and will present data from the European Biomed stroke project to illustrate the potential uses and limitations of such measures.

Subjective outcomes are those which seek to capture the patient's own perspective of aspects of their disease or health status. In this they differ from measures which can be 'objectively' assessed by a professional observer. Subjective outcomes are assumed to be measures of factors which are important to the patient. Their increased use in healthcare evaluation has been attributed to a growing recognition of the need to complement bio-medically defined outcomes with measures that take into account patients' own concerns.[1]

Measurement of patient outcomes is essential for quality assurance of care, investigations of the effectiveness of new methods of treating or caring for patients, and investigation of the efficiency of resource use. The growing interest in outcome measurement throughout Europe reflects a general concern with quality, drives to reform the delivery of healthcare in both Western and Eastern Europe, and the general need for cost containment in the provision of healthcare. Different types of outcome are of interest to different groups, including patients themselves, clinicians, politicians and planners.[2] In a medically focused framework of health interventions, patient outcomes can be narrowly conceptualised as clinical indicators, including mortality, the presence, absence, decrease or increase in pathology, and functional capacity and performance. Mortality data are readily available, but are of little use when assessing the impact of chronic disorder on survivors. For this task, morbidity data are required. However, the definition of morbidity is problematic, and therefore its measurement is not straightforward. Many patient outcome indicators can be objectively measured by the health professional or researcher, including death, coexisting disease and risk factors, although many such measures are subject to the vagaries of inter-rater variation.[3] Subjective outcomes are therefore routinely incorporated into outcome studies as a way of complementing other indicators, to gain a more complete picture of the impact of a condition or an intervention.

In a research paradigm where objective measurement represents a gold standard of data collection, the notion of collecting subjective data may seem paradoxical if not actually unscientific. However, the term 'subjective' here refers to the perception of the patient (the research subject), and may well be something which is not directly observable or measurable. Moreover, the inclusion of patients' perceptions in the overall evaluation of healthcare delivery is useful for a number of reasons. Individuals' decisions about whether to consult doctors in the first place and whether to follow doctors' advice and prescriptions depend on their own perceptions of their health status.[4] Subjectively defined health status has also been shown to predict outcome.[5] In the clinical setting, achieving agreement between patient and professional about behaviour necessary to prevent disease and about therapeutic compliance has long been regarded as problematic. As Kleinman *et al.*[6] have argued, the therapeutic relationship is enhanced when each party understands the perspective of the other. Similarly, in the evaluation of interventions, it is not sufficient to demonstrate the clinical efficacy and cost-effectiveness of a particular method of healthcare delivery – it must also be shown to be acceptable to patients.

Bowling[3] has attributed the increasing popularity of subjective outcome measurement to a number of factors, including the transformed concept of health (which according to the World Health Organisation definition incorporates not just an absence of disease but a more broadly conceptualised 'well-being'), the recognition of the importance of patient satisfaction and how patients feel rather than what statistics tell them they ought to feel, and an increased concern about the management of chronic disease, where the possibility of cure is reduced, and care aims to alleviate symptoms partially or temporarily, and to provide the conditions whereby a comfortable, functional and satisfying life can be achieved.

Box 7.1 Why measure subjective outcomes?

• Individuals' perceptions of their own health or illness influence their use of health services.

Cont

- Individuals' perceptions of their own health or illness influence their relationship with health providers and their decisions about whether to adhere to professional advice.
- Subjectively defined health status is related to clinical outcome.
- Evaluation of services should include evaluation of acceptability to patients.
- Management of chronic disease should aim to achieve a state which is acceptable to the patient.

One of the problems associated with this area is the confusion caused by the terms currently used. Fitzpatrick *et al.*[1] list quality of life, health-related quality of life, health status, functional status and subjective health status under the rubric of healthcare outcomes assessed from the patient's perspective. These terms are not all synonymous, but they do overlap. It is therefore important to be clear about the way in which particular terms are being used. Building on our experience of identifying appropriate measures for the Biomed II stroke study, this chapter will consider the following patient-based outcomes – disability, handicap, and quality of life – all of which can be regarded as components of the broad category of subjective health status. In addition, we consider patient satisfaction, an outcome which does not necessarily reflect health status, but which is important in the evaluation of interventions. Impairment is only briefly dealt with in this chapter, since this is considered to be an objective rather than a subjective outcome. Other subjective outcomes, such as psychological well-being and life satisfaction, are also beyond the scope of this chapter.

Table 7.1   Categories of subjective outcomes

Category	Example of instrument
Disability/functional ability/activities of daily living	Barthel Index
Self-perceived health status	SF-36*
Quality of life/health-related quality of life	WHOQOL**
Handicap	London Handicap Scale
Psychological well-being	General Health Questionnaire
Satisfaction	Carer Hospsat and Homesat

* Short Form 36.
** World Health Organisation Quality of Life.

The ICIDH model

Patient-based outcomes generally aim to assess particular areas of disease consequence as defined by the International Classification of Impairments, Disabilities and Handicaps (ICIDH).[7] Impairment refers to the actual pathology, disability refers to the functional results of impairment, and handicap refers to the social consequences of the disease. Although these three areas are considered to be related in a hierarchical way,[8] the relationship between them is not a simple or necessarily a direct one. Writing of stroke in particular, Ebrahim and Harwood[9] point out that impairment, disability and handicap are the three broad elements which constitute the 'severity' of a stroke, but that each of them can be influenced by a number of factors. Therefore it is important to measure each level separately.[10] These three elements also represent different perspectives, with impairment being of greater concern to clinicians and handicap being of greater concern to patients and their families. The importance of these different realms of disease impact will vary at different stages of the disease process. Measurement of impairment is important at the onset and early stages of the disease to inform a diagnosis and treatment decision making, as well as prognosis. After the acute stage of the disease, when clinical management has been established, the measurement of disability and handicap acquire more significance in terms of assisting the patient to adjust to life with an ongoing disorder and possible limitations to their abilities and lifestyle which may arise as a consequence.

The ICIDH has been undergoing conceptual redevelopment. The new framework 'reflects the model of human functioning in which functioning and disablement are viewed as outcomes of an interaction between a person's physical or mental condition and their social and physical environment'.[11] The levels of functioning have therefore been defined as impairment, activity (a person's daily activities) and participation (which ranges from personal maintenance to social relationships and civic and community life). Among the advantages of the revised classification which its developers have identified are the facts that it is universally applicable, it is based on a social model of functioning and disablement, and it includes environmental barriers and facilitators to participation.

Measuring disability and handicap

The most commonly used measure of disability for stroke patients is the Barthel Index, which was first developed in 1965.[12] It measures performance of everyday tasks related to self-care (feeding, grooming, bathing, dressing and toileting) and mobility (walking, transfers and stair climbing), capturing what have been called *basic activities of daily living*.[13] The Barthel

Index has been shown in a number of studies to be reliable.[14] However, it has also been shown to underestimate the impact of stroke, particularly on those with mild disease.[15]

Other measures, such as the Frenchay Index, are used to assess ability to perform other tasks (*instrumental activities of daily living*), such as leisure and social activities.

The most commonly used measure of 'handicap' in stroke care and research is the Rankin scale, which was first developed in the late 1950s. Scoring requires an assessment of the patient's independence/degree of dependence and the restrictions on their lifestyle which limitations on independence would impose. However, it has also been argued that the Rankin scale does not in fact measure 'handicap' at all, but rather reflects disability.[16] This is attributed to lack of conceptual clarity about handicap itself, with the ICDH indicators of handicap defined in relation to functional abilities and activities, rather than in relation to an individual's circum-stances and social situation. According to Wade[17], measurement of handicap is problematic for a number of reasons. Since it must be assessed by reference to culturally based expectations, there is no absolute standard against which to judge it. Furthermore, because it arises from the interaction between dis-ability and environment, measurement of handicap also requires a measure-ment of the environment, and finally it cannot be directly observed. de Haan *et al.* also suggest that, given these difficulties, 'physicians should not generally focus on handicap as a primary outcome but on a more tangible manifestation of disease in terms of disability'.[16]

Neither the Barthel Index nor the Rankin scale require the patient to respond, but assessment can be made by observation alone by another person, be they a doctor, nurse or family member. This raises the question of whether these measures, when performed by proxy, can properly be described as subjective outcomes.

Quality of life

Quality-of-life assessment is widely regarded as appropriate in the evalua-tion of treatment outcomes and organisation of healthcare services, and in the monitoring and audit of services. There has been enormous growth in quality-of-life research, with measures being adapted, tested and translated into new language versions, and new instruments being developed for specific diseases or conditions. Despite this, there is universal acknowledge-ment of the 'lack of clarity or consistency about the meaning and measure-ment of quality of life'.[18] Perhaps as a consequence of this conceptual confusion, some authors simply avoid defining what they mean by 'quality of life'. Others have called for greater precision in terminology, arguing that where the term *quality of life* is used in a medical context, it should refer only to *health-related quality of life*, and not to more abstract concepts (e.g. life satisfaction) or to non-clinical matters (e.g. living standards).[4,19]

Thus quality of life is problematic as a concept, since it is loose, poorly defined and has been used in different ways by different people. Although it is generally agreed that measurement of quality of life is important as a means of incorporating the patient's perspective on the consequences of disease and treatment,[20] this is not yet routinely performed. In a review of outcome measures used in 174 acute stroke trials, only 2% of studies measured handicap or quality of life, a failing which was attributed to lack of clarity about what these domains mean and how to measure them.[10]

Nevertheless, certain aspects of the consequences of disease are also generally agreed to be important in the assessment of quality of life. According to de Haan *et al.*,[8] writing of the case of stroke in particular, these are physical health, functional health, psychological health and social health. They define these dimensions as follows: 'The physical health dimension refers primarily to disease-related and treatment-related symptoms. Functional health comprises self-care, mobility, and physical activity level, as well as the capacity to carry out various roles in relation to family and work. Cognitive functioning, emotional status (especially post-stroke depression) and general perceptions of health, well-being, life satisfaction and happiness are the central components of the psychological life domain. Social functioning includes the assessment of qualitative and quantitative aspects of social contacts and interactions.' These four dimensions clearly cover a broad range of issues, raising the question of whether quality of life is being measured if all of these aspects are not investigated. Wilkinson *et al.*[21] suggested that, for a group of long-term stroke survivors, the Barthel Index may be a proxy for different outcome measures intended for the assessment of other domains.

Measuring quality of life

Numerous questionnaires have been developed to measure quality of life. These include both generic measures applicable to general populations and disease-specific measures. Generic measures have the disadvantage that the domains which they assess may not be relevant to the particular symptoms of a given disorder, such as stroke. Generic measures which have been used with stroke patients include the SF-36, Euroqol and Sickness Impact Profile (SIP), although some would argue that these are health-status measures and that they do not encompass all of the relevant dimensions of quality of life.

Stroke-specific quality-of-life measures have also recently been developed in the USA,[22,23] but it is still too soon to say whether these will gain wide acceptance. The choice of which quality-of-life instruments to use depends on the purpose of the research, the resources available to conduct the research (e.g. how many interviewing hours are available) and decisions about how much time can be requested of patients and their family members. Some quality-of-life measures, such as the SIP, are rather lengthy, and consideration should be given to the inconvenience which protracted interviewing may represent to patients.

Patient satisfaction

Patient satisfaction is another outcome which has been increasingly incorporated into evaluations of healthcare. The development of patient satisfaction as an outcome in healthcare evaluation is linked to sociological concern with patient–professional relationships, increased pressure to seek the views of patients when monitoring and improving the quality of services, and the shift towards reconceptualising patients as 'consumers'. According to the authors of a recent review, patient satisfaction is measured for three reasons – to describe healthcare from the patient's point of view, as a measure of process of care, and to inform the evaluation of healthcare.[24] Despite the rapid growth in the measurement of patient satisfaction, a number of problems remain unresolved. Little attention has been paid to the meaning of the concept itself.[24,25] This is an important consideration because there is evidence that responses to satisfaction questionnaires may be determined by factors other than the quality of a service. These include patients' expectations, patient characteristics (some studies show that older people are more likely to express satisfaction than younger individuals),[24] and patient psychosocial factors related to the experience of seeking and receiving healthcare or social care.

The broad components of satisfaction have been identified as accessibility to care, interpersonal aspects of care (including empathy and communication), technical aspects of care, and patient information and education. A major weakness identified here is that taxonomies of components of satisfaction tend to be defined by managers and professionals, and thus may not adequately reflect the concerns of patients themselves. However, it is feasible to ensure that questionnaires which are developed reflect lay people's concerns. In the UK, questionnaires were developed to measure satisfaction of stroke patients and their carers with hospital and community services.[26] Qualitative research methods were used to elicit the concerns of patients and to incorporate these in the questionnaires.

Subjective outcome assessment in practice: dilemmas and dangers

It is clear that much work remains to be done in refining the concepts of subjective outcomes such as handicap and quality of life. In the meantime, however, clinicians and policy makers need to be able to have confidence that the measures being used accurately reflect patients' experiences and views. Jenkinson[27] has highlighted the possible danger of inappropriately used measures influencing decision making. Recent research reports illustrate particular problems associated with the imperative to measure subjective outcomes prevailing over our present ability to capture these in a meaningful or sophisticated way. For example, a recently published trial designed to evaluate community support for stroke patients who had been discharged home concluded that there were no differences in physical outcome between the two groups of patients and their carers.[28] Although carer psychosocial outcomes and carer and patient satisfaction were greater in the experimental group than in the control group, the intervention was deemed to have failed, and funding of the service was withdrawn. However, as a number of correspondents to the *British Medical Journal* commented, the generic outcome measures that were used may not have been sensitive enough to detect small changes in a stroke population. This illustrated the possibility that although it may be considered politically important to elicit patients' views, they may count for little when compared with other 'harder' outcomes. Another recent study designed to compare two quality-of-life measures concluded by recommending the tool which yielded a better response rate, without considering how well either instrument reflected the patients' own concerns.[29]

Cross-national studies including patient outcomes

As we have seen, there is a drive towards comparing outcomes cross-nationally. This can be related to several different factors including, in the European context, the wider moves towards harmonisation within the region, the World Health Organisation's goal of 'Health for All', and the globalisation of markets targeted by multinational pharmaceutical companies. In all cases there is a need for indicators which are equally meaningful across countries, so that questions may be expected to elicit the same types of responses. However, there are a number of difficulties in comparing patient outcomes across countries.

In 1977, the adoption by WHO members of 'Health for All' committed member states of WHO Europe to use appropriate indicators to measure progress in achieving health for all targets. However, cross-national comparisons were hampered by the differences in indicators collected in different countries, prompting the European Regional Office to establish a series of international consultations to develop common methods and instruments. WHO Europe acknowledged that this process of harmonisation would be difficult and time consuming.[30] Scientists and pharmaceutical companies conducting international clinical trials are also concerned to use quality-of-life outcome measures as a means of assessing the perceived efficacy and acceptability of particular interventions. Work to date has proceeded according to three diverse strategies. First, measures developed in one setting have been translated and adapted for use in other settings (e.g. SF-36). Secondly, measures have been developed centrally by international teams of experts (e.g. Euroqol). Finally, measures have been developed by following parallel multicentre investigations (e.g. WHOQOL). Translation of existing validated questionnaires would appear to be an efficient method of producing questionnaires for use in countries other than those in which they were originally developed. A number of researchers have described the procedures involved in translation of instruments, and guidelines have been produced.[31] However, methods which begin with investigation of the concepts underpinning the factors to be measured might be theoretically superior. The difficulties associated with quantifying quality of life across different countries and cultures are not only methodological but also conceptual. As anthropologists have long recognised, health and disease are not simply biological entities, but also cultural ones – that is, recognition of diseases, responses to them and meanings attributed to them may vary from one cultural group to another. Such variations lead to differences in factors such as perceptions of health and sickness, the interpretation of symptoms, the meaning of quality of life and expectations for care. These must be understood in order to define and assess quality of life adequately in cross-national studies.[32] Even with a narrow definition of quality of life as *health related*, insufficient attention has been paid to the question of universality of domains attributed to the latter, or to the place of culture in the development of instruments, which should themselves be regarded as culture laden rather than value free.[33] It is unclear how burgeoning international concepts of quality of life and a globally accepted drive to quantify it in healthcare evaluation relate to local systems of knowledge and practice (cf. Good[34]).

Cultural issues also need to be considered in relation to methods of collecting and eliciting information. Are written, telephone or face-to-face questionnaires most appropriate? Different historical situations may have produced variations in the acceptability to patients of being asked certain types of questions. Will respondents simply give the answers which they believe are expected of them by 'officials' such as health researchers?

There appears to have been little research comparing patient satisfaction with interventions cross-nationally. However, the need to compare this outcome across Europe has been assumed by WHO Europe in the targets set as part of the 'Health for All' programme. For example, the target of cost-effective and equitable management of health service resources, secondary and tertiary care and general quality of care all rely on setting and achieving outcome targets, including patient satisfaction. Although this does not necessarily imply the development of a cross-national measure of satisfaction, it does require comparability of indices of satisfaction. However, this would necessitate greater conceptual clarity about what constitutes 'satisfaction' and how the expectations and willingness to express dissatisfaction differ cross-culturally.

The Biomed stroke study experience

Our experience of incorporating subjective outcomes into the data collection conducted for the Biomed stroke study is instructive. We were aware at the outset of the importance of including such measures, and we aimed to collect quality-of-life data as a way of comparing patients' perspectives across different settings. However, we were less aware of the obstacles that we faced.

The first question we considered was whether to use a generic measure of quality of life or a measure specific to stroke disease. Since the study was comparing the same disease outcomes across different care packages and social contexts, it made sense to use a disease-specific measure. However, there was no generally accepted quality-of-life measure specific to stroke disease, although many different generic measures have been used,[8] and since the outset of the study other stroke-specific measures have been developed.[22] Of the generic measures which have been used in studies involving patients with stroke, no instrument was available in all of the language versions that we required. Developing a new measure was well beyond the resources of the project. Adapting an existing measure for use in countries where no approved translation was available was also beyond the scope of the project. This would have been an expensive and time-consuming project in its own right, requiring sophisticated translation procedures and testing of the instrument's psychometric performance.[35] A further difficulty was the fact that only a minority of the researchers involved in the study (most of whom were clinicians rather than full-time researchers) had previous experience of quality-of-life data collection. A great deal of time and resources had already been expended in agreeing upon clinical data-collection items (see Chapter 2) – that is, from those indicators with which the researchers were already familiar. We therefore limited subjective assessment to what could be feasibly achieved. We collected data on functional health status as measured by the Barthel Index and, on an experimental basis, included the 'two simple questions' which were also developed to measure functional outcome. In addition, we hoped to undertake qualitative research into patients' perceptions of the impact of stroke in different settings.

Two simple questions

The 'two simple questions' were developed by Lindley et al.[36] to meet the need for a simple, inexpensive and quick way of assessing functional outcome in large numbers of stroke patients recruited to an open randomised controlled trial. The questions (see Box 7.2) were designed to investigate 'dependency' and 'recovery.' The authors found that these questions provided a valid and reliable assessment of outcome after stroke, they could be administered in a number of ways and they had the advantage of being easily understood both by professionals and by patients and carers.[36,37]

Box 7.2   Two simple questions

• To investigate dependency:

Have you required assistance with everyday activities over the last 2 weeks?

• To investigate recovery:

Do you feel that you have made a complete recovery from stroke?

The two simple questions were included in the Biomed II stroke study questionnaire and asked at 3 and 12 months post stroke. They were translated from English into the appropriate language by each local research co-ordinator, although researchers in the co-ordinating centre were unable to monitor the quality of the translations. To investigate how successfully the two simple questions captured patients' perceptions of recovery and dependence, we assessed the questions' sensitivity (i.e. how well a question identifies all of the positive cases) and specificity (i.e. how well a question identifies all of the negative cases) using 3-month responses from eight participating centres. We used the Barthel Index scores as a 'gold standard'. To analyse responses to the dependency question, we first defined independence as a score of 20 on the Barthel Index, and defined dependence as a Barthel Index score of less than 20. To analyse responses to the recovery question, patients who were classifiable as recovered from stroke were defined as those who had a 3-month Barthel Index score the same as (or better than) their pre-stroke Barthel Index score. Patients classifiable as not recovered were defined as those whose pre-stroke Barthel Index score was greater than their 3-month Barthel Index score.

The question investigating dependency had high sensitivity and specificity. The question investigating recovery also had high specificity, but it had low sensitivity. Therefore the dependency question appeared to capture the same domains as were measured by the Barthel Index. However, the recovery question was not able to identify all those who had a Barthel Index of 20 (i.e. the 'functionally independent'), since 'recovery' is clearly more than the ability to perform the tasks measured by the Barthel Index. There were only minor variations in sensitivity and specificity across centres, which justified its use.

We then compared outcomes across centres. First, we used the algorithm developed during the testing of the two simple questions[36] to identify three outcome groups. Poor outcome was defined as a positive response to the dependency question. Indifferent outcome was defined as a negative response to both the dependency and recovery questions. A good outcome was defined as a positive response to the recovery question. Using multiple logistic regression analysis, we predicted the percentages of responders

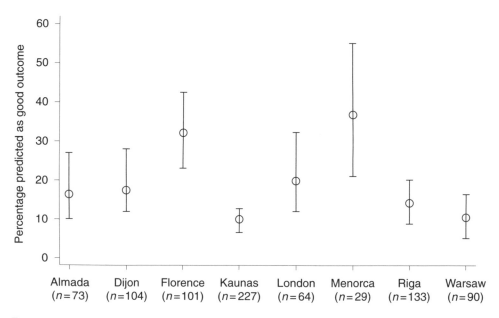

Figure 7.1 Predicted good outcome with 95% confidence intervals for each centre.

(alive at 3 months) who would have a good outcome, adjusting for case mix (age, sex, and for stroke severity urinary incontinence and consciousness level). In order to standardise the case mix across centres, the prediction was made for the average patient. There were variations in outcome as captured by the two simple questions. The percentage of patients with a good outcome ranged from 9.5% in Warsaw and Kaunas to 36.9% in Menorca (*see* Figure 7.1). These may indeed be real differences in outcome. However, there are a number of problems in interpreting these variations. First, the differences could be due to residual case mix differences that were not controlled for in the model. They may reflect respondents' expectations of what constitutes 'recovery' after stroke and their expectations about needs for assistance (both issues which have not been investigated). Finally, a third caveat relates to the quality of the questionnaire translations from English into local languages. Professional questionnaire translation is of course the ideal, but this was beyond the resources of the project.

Qualitative study of the impact of stroke in different settings

'Measuring' quality of life was hampered by the lack of a common tool, lack of a shared conceptual understanding, and the different levels of experience of collecting such data. As an alternative strategy to measurement of quality of life, we undertook qualitative work in selected centres in Western and Eastern Europe with the aim of exploring how patients themselves felt that stroke affected their own lives, and whether perceptions differed across centres with regard to the impact of stroke on their lives. In-depth interviews were conducted with small samples of patients in London, UK and Riga, Latvia, and the interviews were tape-recorded, transcribed in full and analysed for emerging themes. Important issues that were raised included individual and social expectations about the ageing process and social roles of older people, the power of disability to cause changes in social roles and social contacts, the use of personal and social histories to contextualise the illness experience, religious and spiritual concerns, and individual and cross-national variations in access to rehabilitation and social and medical care.

This research indicated that it is possible to compare subjective experiences and expectations of stroke patients in culturally and historically diverse centres. The work also provided contextual data for the quantified outcomes that were being collected in the main body of the study, and offered a useful patient perspective to balance the professional perspective of the study. There were certain pragmatic problems which made it difficult to integrate the qualitative approach into the main study. These were related to the fact that the qualitative approach had not originally been planned, but was added to the methods at a later stage. Therefore the financial and temporal resources available were limited. In addition, it was difficult to make contact with suitable researchers in other centres where collaboration between clinical/epidemiological researchers and social scientists is less well established.

Conclusions

- There are variations in subjective outcomes after stroke across Europe.
- However, we do not understand why this is so. Perhaps part of the problem is that the meaning of the questions remains unclear.
- In-depth studies also highlight cultural differences between countries with regard to quality of life after stroke.

There has been a great deal of work in the field of patient-based outcomes, but much of this has been concerned with psychometric validity. More research needs to be done to investigate the conceptual basis of subjective outcome assessment and the ethical implications of such work. Where policy decisions informed by subjective outcome assessments are made, particular care needs to be taken when interpreting the results obtained by instruments which are at best crude.

Information is available from published literature reviews (*see*, for example, Fitzpatrick *et al.*[1]), networks of researchers in this field (e.g. International Quality of Life Assessment Project – IQOLA) and clearing houses (UK Outcomes Clearing House, and the European Clearing Houses on Health Outcomes – ECHHO, both of which are based at the Nuffield Institute for Health, University of Leeds, UK). However, at a local level, clinicians should be encouraged to make contact with social scientists in university departments to find out about local expertise in this area and promote collaboration between the two disciplines.

Note: Some of the findings in this chapter were published in McKevitt C, Dundas R and Wolfe C (2001) Two simple questions to assess outcome: a European Study. *Stroke.* **32**: 681–6.

References

1 Fitzpatrick R, Davey C, Buxton M and Joens D (1998) Evaluating patient-based outcome measures for use in clinical trials. *Health Technol Assess.* **2**: 14 (review).

2   Stojcevic N, Wilkinson P and Wolfe C (1996) Outcome measures in stroke patients. In: C Wolfe, T Rudd and R Beech (eds) *Stroke Services and Research.* The Stroke Association, London, 261–80.

3   Bowling A (1995) *Measuring Disease.* Open University Press, Milton Keynes.

4   Leplege A and Hunt S (1997) The problem of quality of life in medicine. *JAMA.* **278**: 47–50.

5   Mossey JM and Shapiro E (1982) Self-rated health: a predictor of mortality among the elderly. *Am J Pub Health.* **72**: 800–8.

6   Kleinman A, Eisenberg L and Good B (1988) Culture, illness and care: clinical lessons from anthropologic and cross-cultural research. *Ann Intern Med.* **88**: 251–8.

7   World Health Organisation (1980) *International Classification of Impairments, Disabilities and Handicaps.* WHO, Geneva.

8   de Haan R, Horn J, Limburg M, Van Der Meulen J and Bossuyt P (1993) A comparison of five stroke scales with measures of disability, handicap and quality of life. *Stroke.* **24**: 1178–81.

9   Ebrahim S and Harwood R (1999) *Stroke: epidemiology, evidence and clinical practice.* Oxford University Press, Oxford.

10 Roberts L and Counsell C (1998) Assessment of clinical outcomes in acute stroke trials. *Stroke.* **29**: 986–91.

11 World Health Organisation (1998) *Towards a Common Language for Disablement: ICIDH. The international classification of impairments, activities and participation.* World Health Organisation, Geneva.

12 Mahoney F and Barthel D (1965) Functional evaluation: the Barthel Index. *Maryland State Med J.* **14**: 61–5.

13 Kelly-Hayes M, Robertson JT, Broderick JP *et al.* (1998) The American Heart Association stroke outcome classification. *Stroke.* **29**: 1274–80.

14 D'Olhaberriague L, Litvan I, Mitsias P and Mansbach HH (1996) A reappraisal of reliability and validity studies in stroke. *Stroke.* **27**: 2331–6.

15 Duncan PW, Samsa GP, Weinberger M *et al.* (1997) Health status of individuals with mild stroke. *Stroke.* **28**: 740–5.

16 de Haan R, Limburg M, Bossuyt P, van der Meulen J and Aaronson N (1995) The clinical meaning of Rankin 'handicap' grades after stroke. *Stroke.* **26**: 2027–30.

17 Wade DT (1992) *Measurement in Neurological Rehabilitation.* Oxford University Press, Oxford.

18 Gill TM and Feinstein AR (1994) A critical appraisal of the quality of quality-of-life measurements. *JAMA.* **272**: 619–26.

19 Fitzpatrick R, Fletcher A, Gore S *et al.* (1992) Quality of life measures in health care. *BMJ.* **305**: 1074–7.

20 Meredith P (1996) But was the operation worth it? The limitations of quality of life and patient satisfaction research in healthcare outcome assessment. *J Qual Clin Pract.* **16**: 75–85.

21 Wilkinson P, Wolfe C, Warburton F *et al.* (1997) A long-term follow-up of stroke patients. *Stroke,* **28**: 507–12.

22 Duncan PW, Wallace D, Lai SM, Johnson D, Embretson S and Laster LJ (1999) The Stroke Impact Scale Version 2.0: evaluation of reliability, validity and sensitivity to change. *Stroke.* **30**: 2131–40.

23 Williams LS, Weinberger M, Harris LE, Clark DO and Biller J (1999) Development of a stroke-specific quality-of-life scale. *Stroke.* **30**: 1362–9.

24 Sitzia J and Wood N (1997) Patient satisfaction: a review of issues and concepts. *Soc Sci Med.* **45**: 1829–43.

25 Avis M, Bond M and Arthur A (1995) Satisfying solutions? A review of some unresolved issues in the measurement of patient satisfaction. *J Adv Nurs.* **22**: 316–22.

26 Pound P, Gompertz P and Ebrahim S (1993) Development and results of a questionnaire to measure carer satisfaction after stroke. *J Epidemiol Commun Health.* **47**: 500–5.

27 Jenkinson C (1995) Evaluating the efficacy of medical treatment: possibilities and limitations. *Soc Sci Med.* **41**: 1395–401.

28 Dennis M, O'Rourke S, Slattery J, Staniforth T and Warlow C (1997) Evaluation of a stroke family care worker: results of a randomised controlled trial. *BMJ.* **314**: 1071–7.

29 Dorman PJ, Slattery J, Farrell B and Dennis MS (1997) A randomised comparison of the EuroQol and Short Form-36 after stroke. *BMJ.* **315**: 461.

30 de Bruin A, Picavet HS and Nossikov A (1996) Health interview surveys. Towards international harmonization of methods and instruments. *WHO Reg Publ Eur Ser.* **58**, i–xiii, 1–161.

31 Guillemin F, Bombardier C and Beaton D (1993) Cross-cultural adaptation of health-related quality of life measures: literature review and proposed guidelines. *J Clin Epidemiol.* **46**: 1417–32.

32 Berzon R, Hays RD and Shumaker SA (1993) International use, application and performance of health-related quality of life instruments. *Qual Life Res.* **2**: 367–8.

33 Fox-Rushby J and Parker M (1995) Culture and the measurement of health related quality of life. *Rev Eur Psychol Appl.* **45**. 257–63.

34 Good M (1995) Cultural studies of biomedicine. *Soc Sci Med.* **41**: 461.

35 Bullinger M, Anderson R, Cella D and Aaronson N (1993) Developing and evaluating cross-cultural instruments from minimum requirements to optimal models. *Qual Life Res.* **2**: 451–9.

36 Lindley R, Waddell F, Livingstone M *et al.* (1994) Can simple questions assess outcome after stroke? *Cerebrovasc Dis.* **4**: 314–24.

37 Dennis M, Wellwood I and Warlow C (1997) Are simple questions measure of outcome after stroke? *Cerebrovasc Dis.* **7**, 22–7.

CHAPTER 8

Costing care across Europe

Richard Grieve, Gerald Haidinger, Ilona Purina and Roger Beech

Introduction

Pressure on healthcare budgets has been growing throughout Europe.[1] The ageing population, uptake of expensive new technology and higher expectations about the quality of the health services provided have fuelled demands.[2] Despite this, the level of public funding available for healthcare has remained generally stable.[3] Given these budget constraints and expanding demands, clinicians and policy makers may be required to prioritise interventions based not just on effectiveness but also on cost-effectiveness.[4] The technique of cost-effectiveness analysis provides a framework for assessing the costs and outcomes of different healthcare programmes. Cost-effectiveness analysis can assist decision makers who are aiming to provide care in the most cost-effective way.

This chapter will:

- describe the cost-effectiveness analysis from an international perspective
- describe the methodologies developed to estimate the cost-effectiveness of stroke care in different countries
- present the cost-effectiveness analysis from the European Biomed stroke programme.

What is cost-effectiveness analysis?

Cost-effectiveness analysis (CEA) is a form of economic evaluation which compares the costs and consequences of two or more alternative healthcare programmes.[5] The consequences may be measured using outcome measures such as life-years gained, functional status, or quality of life. The results section reports the ratio of costs to effects of the alternative programmes (e.g. cost per year of life gained). An example of a CEA conducted in several European countries compared the use of simvastatin (a cholesterol-lowering drug) with placebo for the treatment of patients with pre-existing coronary heart disease.[6] The introduction of the statin led to improved life expectancy at a relatively small additional cost. For 70-year-old men the cost per unit of effectiveness was $3800 per life-year gained. The results of these types of analyses may be combined into a 'league table' ranging from best value (lowest cost per unit of effectiveness) to worst value (highest cost per unit of effectiveness).[7] In a recent UK review of published economic evaluations,[8] the relative cost-effectiveness ratios ranged from £9 to £909 001 per life-year gained. The decision maker may use this information to prioritise the most cost-effective programmes. However, commentators have counselled against priority setting on the basis of the results of league tables for a variety of reasons, including differences in methodology[9] and the need to consider other objectives (e.g. equity and patient choice) when allocating resources.[10]

Cost-effectiveness analysis in an international context

When viewed in an international context the use of cost-effectiveness analysis becomes more problematic. In particular, the question which arises is to what extent the results generated in one country apply to another. The scarcity of cost information and research resources (particularly in areas such as health economics), coupled with the increased requirement for information on cost-effectiveness, may lead to results being directly transferred between different countries. In the earlier example, although the use of simvastatin may be relatively cost-effective in the Scandinavian countries studied, this result may not apply elsewhere because of differences in the baseline effectiveness of existing therapies or differences in the costs of current practice. A recent review of published evaluations of adjuvant therapies for cancer[11] found that none of the 26 published evaluations were applicable to the setting concerned (France).

In order to establish whether costs vary between different countries, methods are needed for measuring the costs of care in different countries in the same way. As part of a Biomed II project a standard method was developed for measuring the costs of stroke across Europe.

Box 8.1   The needs for methods to assess cross-country cost variability

- European governments are faced with spiralling costs and limited healthcare budgets.

Cont

- CEA can provide information on the relative cost-effectiveness of competing interventions.
- The extent to which results generated in one country are applicable to another may be limited by a number of factors, including cross-country cost variability.
- Standard methods for assessing cross-country cost variability would enable the extent to which costs vary across countries to be assessed.

The Biomed II stroke study as a case study illustrating a standard costing method

Rationale

The Biomed II stroke study is used as a case study to illustrate the potential of developing a standard method to examine the reason for cost variability across different European centres. Stroke consumes a high proportion of healthcare resources,[12] so it is important to manage the disease in a cost-effective way. A recent review[13] found that previous costing work has focused on calculating the total costs of stroke using a highly aggregated approach to costing. Differences in the methodologies used in the various studies hindered any attempts to compare the costs of different ways of managing stroke.

Costing methodology

A standard costing method was developed which incorporated general guidelines on measuring costs in economic evaluation.[14,15] This meant that a four-stage process of cost measurement was embarked upon. First, a common list of resource use items likely to be important for comparing the costs of acute stroke was agreed upon. Secondly, the level of resource use (e.g. number of CT scans) was measured. Thirdly, a unit cost for each centre (e.g. cost of a CT scan) was assigned, and fourthly, resource use was multiplied by the relevant unit cost to give a total cost per case. At each stage, comparisons between the centres were made in order to investigate whether differences in resource use or unit cost were important in explaining any differences in total cost.

Apart from following this general guidance for costing work within a national healthcare system, certain methodological features were incorporated to take into account the international nature of the work and enable the reasons for the cost variability to be explored. These are set out below.

Broad perspective

To allow for differences in the structures of the healthcare systems, it was important to take a broad approach to cost measurement. This meant that care provided in different settings was included in the analysis (primary, secondary and ambulatory care, and by patients and their carers). The enormity of this task meant that the work was carried out in two phases. Phase 1 involved measuring the resource use and costs in the acute hospital, and in phase 2 all costs incurred post discharge were included, covering the whole spectrum of health, community and personal health services. Importantly, care financed by general taxation (or social insurance), private insurance or out-of-pocket payments was included in the analysis.

Prospective patient-based study

Patients were prospectively recruited to the study, which enabled standard inclusion and exclusion criteria, measures of resource use and measures of case severity to be used. Questionnaires were administered to record items of resource use (e.g. number of GP visits which would not have been routinely available). By measuring resource use and unit costs for each patient, it was possible to use standard statistical techniques to compare costs between the centres, adjusting for any case-mix differences.

Inclusion and exclusion criteria

The centres included were in the UK, Austria, Germany, Denmark, France, Spain, Portugal, Hungary, Poland, Latvia and Lithuania. Although the selected centres may not be representative of the stroke services provided in each country, each hospital provides general acute care for the local population. Consecutive stroke patients (defined using the WHO criteria) who were admitted to hospital during 1996–97 were included in the study, and patients with subarachnoid haemorrhage were excluded.

Case-mix measurement

Information was collected on age, sex, urinary incontinence and level of consciousness at the time of maximum impairment (subsequently dichoto-mised into coma and non-coma).[16] These measures of case severity have been shown to be associated with differences in cost.[17]

Box 8.2   Key features of the method

* Broad perspective
* Prospective study
* Standard inclusion and exclusion criteria
* Same items of resource use measured across centres
* Development of standard method for measuring staff time
* Unit costing carried out using similar framework
* Adjustment for price differences between centres
* Adjustment for case mix and skewness in cost distribution

Resource use measurement

Resource use was recorded for the year following stroke. The first phase of the project covered resource consumption in the acute hospital. The length of stay by ward type and the use of diagnostic investigations was recorded for each patient. One researcher (RG) visited each centre and used a semi-structured questionnaire to record the average time that staff spent with stroke patients. The aim was to measure in a consistent way the time for which each professional group was available to provide services for stroke patients, so that the average staff time per occupied bed day could be compared across the centres.

In phase 2 the length of stay in rehabilitation hospitals, nursing homes and sheltered homes was again recorded by investigators using standard forms. The use of outpatient services (hospital clinics and therapy services) and community services (GP visits, home helps, meals-on-wheels, home nursing, day hospitals, day centres) was recorded from interviews with the patients and their relatives. In addition, patient and carer resource use (e.g. in taking time off work to visit follow-up clinics, or to prepare meals for the patient) was recorded on the questionnaires.

Costing

The finance departments at each centre provided unit costs which were used to value each item of resource use. For the acute hospital costs the length of stay was multiplied by the relevant unit costs and added to the investigation costs to give a total cost for each patient. For the costs of institutional and community services, interviews were undertaken with a range of providers, and the median cost of the item concerned was used.

The average market wage for the economy concerned was used to value patients' and carers' time.[18] All costs were adjusted to a 1995 price base using the relevant price index.[19]

Adjustment for price differences between the countries concerned

Costs were initially converted from local currencies into dollars using 1995 official exchange rates.[19] However, price differences between countries may not be reflected by market exchange rates.[20] Instead, purchasing power parities (PPP) conversion factors[19] were used to convert the costs from local currencies into dollars (*see* Box 8.3).

Box 8.3   Comparing nursing costs in Germany and Latvia

If the hourly cost of a German nurse is DM 42.67, converting into dollars using the market rate of $1 = 1.67 DM means that the nurse costs *$27.53/hour*. However, the relative price levels in the German economy are higher than indicated by the market exchange rate. To buy 1 dollarsworth of goods takes not 1.67 DM but 2.07 DM. Therefore using the PPP factor ($1 = 2.07 DM) to convert the nursing costs gives a value of *$20.62/hour*.

In Latvia a nurse costs 0.37 Lats/hour. Converting that cost into dollars using the market exchange rates ($1 = 0.50 Lats) gives the cost in dollars as *$0.74/hour*. However, in Latvia 1 dollarsworth of goods can be bought with just 0.30 Lats. Therefore using this PPP factor ($1 = 0.30 Lats) to convert the cost into dollars means that the nursing cost is now *$1.23/hour*.

Thus the difference in nursing costs between Germany and Latvia is less when the conversion is made using the PPP index to take into account general differences in price levels that are not reflected by the market exchange rate.

Adjustment for case-mix differences and skewness in the distribution of costs

The arithmetic mean cost in each centre was calculated for acute hospital costs (phase 1 of the project), and for 3- and 12-month costs (phase 2). Multiple linear regression was performed to investigate the relationship between the log of the total cost and centre, adjusting for age group, gender, consciousness level and incontinence. As the distribution of costs was skewed, the geometric mean cost for treating a reference group (conscious, continent men, aged >74 years) was predicted for each centre from the regression coefficients. The regression analysis was repeated with separate models for those who died in hospital and those who survived.

Results from phase 1: acute hospital costs

A total of 2072 patients were recruited to the study. Of these, 110 patients had missing case-mix variables and were excluded from the analysis. The patient-based method enabled the reasons for between-centre differences in costs to be explored in terms of case mix, duration and intensity of resource use, unit cost and total cost before and after case-mix adjustment. This can be shown by directly comparing the UK and Austrian centres.

Despite the specification of standard inclusion and exclusion criteria, there were general differences between the centres in the case mix of patients recruited to the study. The case mix was more severe in the London centre than in the Austrian centre (see Table 8.1).

The mean length of hospital stay was similar in the UK and Austrian centres (see Table 8.2). However, the limitations of using this aggregate

Table 8.1 Demographic and case-mix characteristics

Country	Number	Mean age years (SD)	Male (%)	Conscious (%)	Continent (%)	Survivors (%)*
Portugal	110	67.7 (12.29)	51	68	52	75
Spain	52	75.2 (8.52)	56	85	50	69
UK	106	73.7 (11.72)	55	79	53	69
Austria	89	69.7 (13.07)	51	94	89	91
France	138	73.2 (17.02)	42	76	67	84
Germany (A)	94	73.3 (12.47)	44	90	74	69
Germany (B)	141	68.8 (13.22)	52	87	52	93
Denmark	318	69.8 (14.06)	50	85	54	84
Hungary	148	62.7 (14.90)	58	79	48	81
Poland	128	72.0 (11.94)	35	88	64	82
Lithuania (A)	84	68.3 (10.87)	37	92	70	85
Lithuania (B)	237	71.6 (11.28)	36	95	62	84
Latvia	317	64.2 (11.41)	49	63	69	66
Total	1962	69.2 (13.31)	47	82	62	79

*Patients who survived the hospital stay.

Table 8.2 Average duration and intensity of resource use

Centre	Length of stay (days)	Brain scans	Doctors' time (minutes/ bed-day)	Nurses' time (minutes/ bed-day)	Therapists' time (minutes/ bed-day)
Portugal	12.1	1.16	99	303	15
Spain	8.8	1.02	43	243	12
UK	35.4	0.94	24	329	56
Austria	31.6	2.35	78	330	69
France	11.5	1.40	30	252	22
Germany (A)	24.4	1.71	55	168	31
Germany (B)	13.9	1.92	99	172	26
Denmark	21.9	1.12	66	239	65
Hungary	26.6	2.28	56	95	24
Poland	22.5	1.20	91	147	32
Lithuania (A)	17.3	0.99	40	196	8
Lithuania (B)	18.1	0.24	22	158	8
Latvia	13.4	1.20	21	57	25

Table 8.3 Costs per hour converted into dollars using the official exchange rate ($) and the purchasing power parity index (PPP $)

Centre	Mid-grade nurse		Mid-grade doctor	
	$	PPP $	$	PPP $
Portugal	12.97	16.41	23.14	29.26
Spain	16.72	17.79	26.60	28.14
UK	21.66	21.66	19.85	19.85
Austria	24.25	18.14	25.59	19.15
France	23.40	19.18	34.21	28.04
Germany (A)	27.45	20.56	33.59	25.14
Germany (B)	27.53	20.62	33.59	25.14
Denmark	27.00	18.21	40.77	27.51
Hungary	3.64	5.62	4.16	6.44
Poland	2.25	3.86	8.74	14.99
Lithuania (A)	0.76	2.16	1.05	3.01
Lithuania (B)	1.03	2.95	0.88	2.51
Latvia	0.82	1.37	1.12	1.87

marker of resource utilisation may be shown by considering the relative intensity of resource use. For example, the use of brain scans, Doppler investigations and doctors' time were higher in the Austrian centre.

The relative impact of unit costs depends on the conversion factor used. When the official exchange rate was used, the unit costs of doctors' or nurses' time were higher in Austria than in the UK. However, once adjustment had been made for the relatively higher costs of living in Austria using the PPP index, the unit costs were found to be slightly higher in the UK (*see* Table 8.3).

The mean total acute care costs were $2000 higher in the Austrian centre than in the UK centre. However, just using this aggregated comparison offers no insight into the reasons for the differences in costs (e.g. differences in treatment intensity), and the potential implications for quality of care and outcome.

Finally, the results from the linear regression analysis (*see* Table 8.4) demonstrated that after adjusting for case mix and skewness in the distribution of costs, differences between the centres remained. In the direct comparison of London and Austria, the less severe case mix in Austria means that this centre still costs more than the London centre after these adjustments have been made.

Table 8.4   Predicted mean total cost (95% CI) ($ PPP) of treating men aged >74 years who were conscious and continent, in each centre*

Country	Whole sample (n = 1962)	Survivors (n = 1554)	Died in hospital (n = 408)
Portugal	2056 (1646–2567)	2113 (1748–2555)	1589 (655–3855)
Spain	1161 (849–1588)	1191 (915–1551)	1693 (857–3344)
UK	3317 (2678–4107)	3250 (2698–3916)	7519 (2674–21138)
Austria	5164 (4294–6211)	5202 (4423–6120)	6191 (2737–14004)
France	1522 (1277–1815)	1547 (1330–1801)	808 (181–3596)
Germany (A)	4072 (3338–4967)	4259 (3534–5132)	3331 (1957–5667)
Germany (B)	2606 (2143–3168)	2640 (2234–3120)	1528 (509–4584)
Denmark	2097 (1824–2409)	2139 (1895–2414)	2538 (1460–4413)
Hungary	979 (802–1196)	1008 (846–1201)	1291 (511–3260)
Poland	1253 (1049–1497)	1267 (1086–1478)	3070 (857–11000)
Lithuania (A)	597 (479–744)	656 (542–794)	129 (36–467)
Lithuania (B)	499 (427–582)	531 (464–608)	134 (52–343)
Latvia	220 (191–254)	240 (210–274)	160 (105–245)

*Results from the multiple regression analysis with log (total cost) as outcome, adjusting for age group, sex, coma and incontinence.

Conclusions

The aim of this case study was to outline a method for measuring costs across European centres which enabled the reasons for the cost differences to be explored. Differences were found between the centres in the intensity of the resources used (e.g. use of doctors' time), the duration of resource use (e.g. length of hospital stay) and the levels of unit cost. This may indicate differences in the quality of care, which may explain previously observed differences in outcomes.[21] Therefore the method outlined may be used to provide further assessment of the quality associated with different ways of providing care. However, firm conclusions about the effects of different models of care on the costs and outcomes cannot be drawn from the phase 1 study because of the narrow perspective taken.[22] For example, care inputs in the rehabilitation hospital, the community or the patient's home have not been included. The phase 2 analysis will include care inputs from a broad range of providers, and will provide a more balanced comparison of the relative costs of the different models of care. Combining these costs with outcomes at 1 year post stroke will enable the relative cost-effectiveness of different models of stroke care to be assessed. Given the observed variations in clinical practice in other clinical areas,[23,24] the method might be useful for investigating the relative cost-effectiveness of different models of care in other disease areas.

Implications for cost-effectiveness analysis

The use of a standard method of cost measurement enabled the costs of stroke to be compared across different settings. This meant that cost variations between countries could be exposed which were not attributable to differences in the methods used. Even from these early results, further doubts were cast on the extent to which the results from economic evaluations performed in one setting can be transferred to another. For example, a drug which improves functional status for a particular client group may enable patients to be discharged earlier. However, the extent to which costs may be saved may vary according to many factors, including the intensity of resource use at the particular centre, and the relative cost-effectiveness of the drug would therefore vary according to the location. The results of economic evaluations may need to be adapted to the local context[25] before they can be used for setting priorities.

The variability of costs across countries also has implications for the methods used in multinational economic evaluations. In these studies, costs are often assumed to be the same in countries with 'similar' healthcare systems.[26] Our study found that even where the health infrastructure was broadly similar, the resource use, unit costs and costs varied between different countries. For example, although the German and French centres show certain similarities in the level of national health infrastructure,[19] it would be inaccurate to assume that the costs of care are the same. Thus, rather than conducting multinational economic evaluations which make inaccurate assumptions, it may be preferable to perform a separate local costing exercise which can capture variability in resource use and unit costs.

Despite the use of standard inclusion and exclusion criteria, the case mix of patients included varied greatly between the centres. The use of a patient-based approach meant that it was possible to utilise regression analysis to adjust for differences in case severity between the centres. The use of this methodology can be recommended for future multicentre costing studies.

Development of local expertise

The process of developing the standard costing method enabled local clinicians to gain an insight into the methods required to perform the costing aspect of an economic evaluation. This could encourage the growth of economic evaluations in the countries concerned and reduce the reliance on results transferred from elsewhere.

Areas for future research

Following on from the development and use of the method outlined in this case study, the following areas would seem to be particularly important for future research.

Assessment of the generalisability of the results from participating centres to other healthcare settings

The centres participating in this study were mainly teaching hospitals, and the costs are unlikely to be representative of the countries concerned. In order to assess the extent to which costs may vary between centres within particular countries, this method could be replicated in various hospitals with different practice patterns and local unit costs.

Testing the applicability of aspects of this method for measuring disease costs to other chronic illnesses

This method has emphasised certain methodological features, such as standard inclusion criteria, the use of recommended case-mix measures, the separate measurement of resource use and cost, and the use of regression analysis to adjust for between-centre case-mix differences. To investigate the importance of applying these methodological features in other disease areas, further primary research is needed. This could help to give general guidance as to when results can be transferred between different countries and when the differences in practice patterns and associated costs mean that the transfer of results would be extremely misleading.

Developing health-specific PPPs which can be used in international costing studies

In this study, general PPPs were used to adjust the cross-centre cost comparisons for differences in the overall price levels in the countries concerned. However, a more accurate comparison would be made if cost comparisons were adjusted for specific differences in the price of healthcare. For these countries, health-specific PPPs were either unavailable or were based on differences in the price of pharmaceuticals which may not represent general price differences in the healthcare sector. Further research is needed to develop these indices.

In conclusion, the method developed as part of the Biomed II stroke study adapted guidance on producing national economic evaluations to an international context. Of particular importance was the use of a prospective patient-based approach to cost measurement which enabled the resources used, unit costs and costs to be compared across countries. The results from the acute costing phase of the work suggest that there is considerable cost variation across Europe. This may have important implications for the transferability of results between different European settings and the methods used in the multinational economic evaluation of healthcare interventions.

Note: Some of the findings in this chapter were published in Grieve R, Dundas R, Beech R and Wolfe CDA (2001) The development and use of a method to compare the costs of acute stroke across Europe. *Age Ageing*. **30**: 67–72.

References

1   Williams C, Coyle D, Gray A *et al.* (1995) European School of Oncology Advisory Report to the Commission of the European Communities for the Europe against Cancer Programme 'Cost-effectiveness in cancer care'. *Eur J Cancer.* **31A**: 1410–24.

2   Schieber G (1995) Preconditions for health reform: experiences from the OECD countries. *Health Policy.* **32**: 279–93.

3   Hurst JW (1991) Reforming health care in seven European Nations. *Health Affairs.* **10**: 8–21.

4   Jonsson E and Banta D (1999) Management of health technologies: an international view. *BMJ.* **319**: 1–3.

5   Drummond MF, O'Brien BJ, Stoddart GL *et al.* (1997) *Methods for the Economic Evaluation of Health Care Programmes* (2e). Oxford University Press, Oxford.

6   Johannesson M, Jonsson B, Kjekshus J *et al.* for the Scandinavian Simvastatin Survival Study Group (1997) Cost-effectiveness of simvastatin treatment to lower cholesterol levels in patients with coronary heart disease. *NEJM.* **336**: 332–6.

7   Williams AH (1984) Economics of coronary artery bypass grafting. *BMJ.* **291**: 326–9.

8   Briggs AH and Gray AM (1999) Handling uncertainty when performing economic evaluation of health care interventions. *Health Technol Assess.* **3**: 4–5.

9   Drummond MF, Torrance GW and Mason J (1993) Cost-effectiveness league tables: more harm than good? *Soc Sci Med.* **37**: 33–40.

10   Klein R, Day P and Redmayne S (1996) *Priority Setting and Rationing in the National Health Service.* Open University Press, Buckingham.

11   Späth HM, Carrère MO, Fervers B and Philip T (1999) Analysis of the eligibility of published economic evaluations for transfer to a given healthcare system. Methodological approach and application to the French healthcare system. *Health Policy.* **49**: 161–77.

12   Isard P and Forbes J (1992) Cost of stroke. *Cerebrovasc Dis.* **2**: 47–50.

13   Porsdal V and Boysen G (1997) Cost-of-illness studies of stroke. *Cerebrovasc Dis.* **7**: 258–63.

14   Drummond MF and Jefferson TO (1996) Guidelines for the authors and peer reviewers of economic submissions to the *BMJ. BMJ.* **313**: 275–83.

15   Gold MR, Siegel JE, Russell LB *et al.* (1996) *Cost-Effectiveness in Health and Medicine.* Oxford University Press, New York.

16   Teasdale G and Jennett B (1974) Assessment of coma and impaired consciousness: a practical scale. *Lancet.* **2**: 81–3.

17   Porsdal V and Boysen G (1999) Costs of health care and social services during the first year after ischaemic stroke. *Int J Technol Assess Health Care.* **15**: 573–84.

18   International Labour Organisation (1998) *Yearbook of Labour Statistics.* International Labour Organisation, Geneva.

19   World Bank (1997) *World Development Report.* World Bank, Washington, DC.

20   Kanavos P and Mossialos E (1999) International comparisons of health care expenditures: what we know and what we do not know. *J Health Serv Res Policy.* **4**: 122–6.

21   Wolfe C, Tilling K, Beech R *et al.* (1999) Variations in case-fatality and dependency from stroke in West and Central Europe. *Stroke.* **30**: 350–6.

22   Byford S and Raftery J (1998) Perspectives in economic evaluation. *BMJ.* **316**: 1529–30.

23   Wennberg JE, Freeman JL and Culp WJ (1985) Are hospital services rationed in New Haven or over-utilised in Boston? *Lancet.* **1**: 1185–9.

24   Anderson TF and Mooney G (1990) *The Challenge of Medical Practice Variations.* Macmillan, Basingstoke.

25   Menzin J, Oster G, Davies L *et al.* (1996) A multinational economic evaluation of rhDNase in the treatment of cystic fibrosis. *Int J Technol Assess Health Care.* **12**: 152–61.

26   Glick H, Wilke R, Polsky D *et al.* (1998) Economic analysis of tirilazad mesylate for aneurysmal subarachnoid hemorrhage. *Int J Technol Assess Health Care.* **14**: 145–60.

CHAPTER 9

Lessons learned

Shah Ebrahim

Preconceptions

If you had to have a stroke, where in Europe would you do best? What is the quality of European stroke services? Does it matter? After all, whatever the quality of services, if you have had a bad stroke you will not do well. These are some of the ideas that went through our minds as we talked about stroke in Europe. Preconceptions about health services are abundant. For example, the British with their 'wonderful' National Health Service are too mean, the Italians have too many doctors and are anarchic, the Germans spend too much money and time correcting every tiny metabolic and electrolyte disturbance, the northern Europeans are too serious and the southern Europeans have more fun. The first lesson we have learned from European collaboration is that our preconceptions are not evidence based, and collecting new evidence to examine quality of healthcare requires all preconceptions to be discarded.

Objectives of healthcare

Quality of healthcare is usually assessed using Donabedian's triad of structure, process and outcome[1] as in this book, although this simple framework is increasingly being reformulated to produce more detailed concepts such as effectiveness, efficiency, appropriateness, humanity and equity.[2] Of these concepts, effectiveness and efficiency are fundamental to any discussion of quality of healthcare. The others are perhaps less obvious. Carotid endarterectomy for high degrees of carotid artery stenosis reduces the risk of future strokes,[3,4] but for smaller stenoses, and as practised in some centres,[5] it is not appropriate. Humane care will involve many common courtesies and respect for the patient's autonomy and dignity. It will also entail providing care in appropriate settings for disabled and often frail people. Equity calls for equal access to treatment for people who do not fit the norm – be they elderly patients, people from black and ethnic minorities, or homeless people.

Using stroke as an illustration of an investigation into the measurement of the quality of healthcare across Europe provides a lens through which our ideas about this common but often forgotten disease can be extended beyond the narrow confines of simply establishing stroke units across the world. If we are to plan and evaluate services for patients who are at risk of or have suffered a stroke, it is helpful to have a framework for thinking about the different functions that health services offer. A simple classification is shown in Box 9.1.

Box 9.1   Objectives of healthcare

- To prevent disease
- To cure disease and its complications
- To increase life expectancy
- To alleviate or palliate distressing symptoms
- To maximise physical and social functioning
- To explain unusual phenomena and offer a prognosis
- To support families and other carers

Source: Ebrahim S and Harwood R (1999) *Stroke: epidemiology, evidence and clinical practice*. Oxford University Press, Oxford.

Stroke care involves all of these objectives. There are now several proven interventions that can decrease the risk of stroke, such as treatment of hypertension and use of anticoagulation or antiplatelet drugs in patients with atrial fibrillation. Stroke complications such as pressure sores and joint contractures can be prevented with appropriate nursing and physiotherapy interventions. Thrombolytic therapy attempts to 'cure' a stroke that would otherwise have evolved, and a few of the rare causes of stroke, such as infective endocarditis, are curable. High-quality stroke care, such as that which is provided on dedicated stroke units, reduces stroke mortality and improves functional outcomes compared with lower-quality care. Stroke patients are prone to pain (e.g. in a subluxing shoulder) and depression, which may both be relieved by treatment. Many stroke manifestations, such as perceptual impairments, are bewildering and require explanation. Recovery from a stroke is often slower than for many other medical conditions, and the risk of recurrence is relatively high, so information on the prognosis is required. Supporting the carers of stroke survivors who remain very dependent is also important if such care is to be maintained for any length of time.

A second lesson we have learned is that we have to ask the right questions. A theoretical understanding of quality of healthcare demonstrates the multidimensional nature of 'quality'. There is no simple answer to the question 'Is this service good or bad?' Rather, the question should be rephrased as a series of questions that, if answered, would provide a comprehensive understanding of what a service is seeking to achieve, whether it is succeeding in achieving its objectives, in part or as a whole, and by what means. It would be surprising for any health service to be completely without value, or indeed to be completely perfect. In attempting to simplify the evaluation of stroke services reported here, sacrifices inevitably have to be made. The focus on structure, process and outcome provides only a partial view of the quality of healthcare that is offered and received.

Observation: defining and finding strokes

Having decided what healthcare is for and how to go about assessing quality, the issue of how best to define a stroke arises. The standard World Health Organisation definition[6] has been used for many years, but it fails to distinguish haemorrhagic from ischaemic stroke, or lacunar from other types of ischaemic stroke. Our understanding of the epidemiology of stroke is badly hampered by our lack of an agreed, widely applicable method of classifying strokes. CT scanning is not a complete answer to the problem, but careful, standardised clinical examination (often repeated), together with neuroradiology, will permit accurate diagnoses of stroke subtype. However, this is difficult to achieve in practice, particularly in poorer countries that lack CT scanners, and for those patients who are being managed at home.

One important key to defining the burden of stroke is knowing where the patients came from — that is, defining the population at risk. In these European studies, we did not attempt to use population laboratories[7] in which accurate censuses and risk factor profiles are available. In many countries of the former Soviet Union and in central Europe where stroke mortality rates appear to be rising, it is apparent that routine reporting of mortality and routine censuses may well be below acceptable levels of accuracy.[8] Nor were we able to monitor all of the strokes arising in such defined populations. Rather, the intensity of ascertainment was very dependent on the resources that the study centre could find to do the job. 'Hot pursuit' (i.e. checking hospital wards daily) as a method of finding strokes is likely to have very different meanings and effects in countries where strokes are managed at home or in hospital with different admission rates for stroke. If more resources had been available, we would have wanted to establish populations at risk and monitor all strokes occurring within these populations using similar staffing levels to ensure an equal ascertainment effort. We would have used capture–recapture methods to obtain estimates of completeness of ascertainment between centres.[9]

Defining the outcomes of health services is also of considerable importance if variations are to be studied. Ensuring that definitions of health states are robust enough to be applied without confusion or bias is fundamental to any study, but becomes more difficult if cross-cultural applicability is required. Even defining death causes problems. What is a stroke death? Is it a death from any cause occurring in a person who has suffered a stroke at some time in the past, and if so, how long ago? Or is it a death due to brain damage from stroke? Or is it a death that occurs within 30 days of a stroke? All of these are perfectly acceptable definitions, but if a consensus is not achieved between study centres, profoundly different patterns of mortality may be found. And if death is a complicated outcome, what of recovery, quality of life and patient satisfaction?

So called 'simple questions' designed to assess recovery (e.g. Have you required assistance with everyday activities over the last 2 weeks? Do you feel that you have made a complete recovery from stroke?)[10] are far from simple when used cross-culturally. They were designed as outcomes for a large randomised trial of aspirin and heparin treatment, in patients with acute stroke, which might reduce brain damage and improve survival and recovery. They were not designed to evaluate complex healthcare systems for stroke patients. The face validity of many health-status measures (e.g. SF-36, EuroQoL, WHOQOL) is poor for examining the effects of services for specific diseases.

Variation in outcomes

In classical epidemiology, describing variation is a crucial step in understanding possible causal mechanisms. Similarly, in health services research, examining the extent of variation in outcomes or service supply is an important step. The twofold variation in probability of death at 3 months following stroke between European study centres raises important questions. For example, is this due to the type of patients or the type of service? Constructing league tables is always popular, but their interpretation is seldom straightforward. Even when careful 'case-mix' adjustment is made using clinical data on stroke severity, no allowance can be made for the biases that result in different types of patients arriving at different hospital services. Examining trends in outcomes over time would be more productive, as most of the case-mix and selection biases will remain the same, particularly over short periods of time, in a single study centre. Enthusiasm for protracted collection of data using comparable methods over a period of several years is limited, but would provide a much better understanding of which services are improving and which are not. Underlying such questions of the quality of a health service is a causal question. What is causing outcomes to vary? This takes us to the next step in epidemiological thinking, namely looking for associations that may be causal.

Association between healthcare and other exposures and outcomes

The methods available for examining the relationship between health service inputs in terms of costs, staff, technology and time fall into two broad groups, namely observational and experimental. In these studies of European centres, the obvious approach was to use observational methods focused on measuring as many aspects of the service, its users and its providers as seemed to be feasible and relevant. Then, the associations between health service input data and health outcomes could be examined. The European studies described here were limited to only a small number of centres. Ideally, a large number of centres within each country would be recruited so that an analysis of healthcare costs, for example, and their relationship with outcomes, could be made both within and between countries. The European studies do show that it is feasible to make cost comparisons between countries, and that outcomes can be measured in comparable ways, but the link between the two remains elusive.

There is considerable enthusiasm and expertise with regard to setting up chronic disease registers, and stroke registers in particular. Such registers often seek to examine the causes of subtypes of stroke, but they never recruit a comparison group in which similar measures of risk factors are made. This was a missed opportunity in our European studies. It would have been perfectly feasible to establish a very large case–control study to examine stroke risk factors, but perhaps not in terms of the available resources.

Causation: randomised comparisons

Defining causal relationships is difficult without experimental methods in which the factors that appear to be of critical importance in observational studies are tested by randomly applying the factor(s) to some patients and not to others. Trials are now much more commonly used in stroke care, and while there is a growing consensus that one element of stroke care, namely organised stroke units (see Figure 9.1), is of benefit,[11] little is known about the cost-effectiveness of such care, or about the efficacy of a wide range of community services for stroke patients or of specific types of rehabilitation. What constitutes 'organised care' remains vague, and it is still unclear which bits work and which do not. The Cochrane Library is an excellent resource,

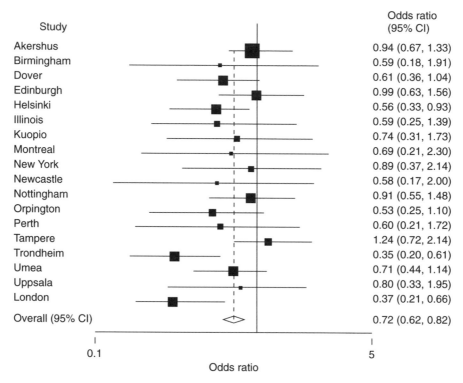

Figure 9.1 Death or dependency at end of follow-up for organised stroke care vs. usual care.[11]

producing systematic reviews of many of these trials, updating them and providing useful pointers for clinical practice and further research. However, it is very unlikely that every intervention received by stroke patients today will be subjected to randomised controlled trial evaluation of its efficacy and cost-effectiveness. Large-scale observational evaluations can provide some pointers to what works, and they should not be disparaged as poor science. Some evaluation is better than none.

Implementation: community effectiveness

The assessment of effectiveness and cost-effectiveness is a major step forward in finding out what works. However, in practice, healthcare is more complicated than a clinical trial. In the real world, some people simply fail to receive effective interventions, some interventions are applied suboptimally and so fail to deliver their full effects, and some patients are unwilling or unable to adhere to treatments[12] (see Figure 9.2). These factors all multiply together to reduce the effects seen in routine clinical practice — sometimes referred to as community effectiveness as distinct from efficacy.

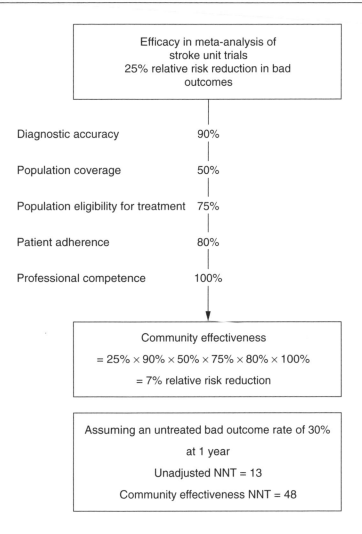

Figure 9.2 The trial efficacy to community effectiveness chain: example drawn from stroke units. NNT = numbers needed to treat.

This chain from population coverage, diagnostic accuracy and professional compliance to patient adherence receives remarkably little attention from researchers, clinicians or public health workers, yet it is a substantial source of lost health gain. Future collaborative European projects might do well to start with an examination of this phenomenon and look at ways in which each link in the chain could be strengthened.

Finally, it is essential that routine evaluation of the community impact of health services is undertaken so that incremental improvements may be made and the place of new technologies understood. Routine evaluation is achieved through monitoring systems, audit and quality control, and involves careful gearing of what is found with systematic feedback and training. In stroke, as in many other areas of clinical practice, only limited routine evaluation is in place, much of which is confined to the hospital sector and little of which is focused on community and primary care services.

Conclusions

Positive outcomes of European research include the following.

- Opportunities exist for EU research.
- Data collection is feasible.
- Good science is feasible.
- Collaboration is stimulating.
- New issues are identified.
- EU findings inform the European debate.

Issues that could be tackled in the future include:

- the broader objectives of healthcare in Europe
- more detailed assessment of quality of care
- more accurate assessment of case mix
- more holistic assessment of outcome
- identification of interventions of specific points of difference in care (e.g. rehabilitation)
- addressing issues to improve efficacy.

Much remains to be done in deciding how best to spend resources on healthcare. Achieving health gain is only part of the equation. Neglected topics include management of the complications of stroke, listening to and providing patients and their carers with what they want, and providing 'dignified' care. Europe-wide collaborations provide a unique means of breaking away from national preconceptions of what is feasible and what 'should' be done. They also provide the only way of examining radically different approaches to the same clinical problem. The methods required are not straightforward, and it is hoped that the material in this book will contribute to the building of further strong European collaborations in the future.

References

1 Donabedian A (1989) The quality of medical care. How can it be assessed? *JAMA*. **260**: 1743–8.
2 Maxwell R (1984) Quality assessment in health care. *BMJ*. **288**: 1470–2.

3   European Carotid Surgery Trialists' Collaborative Group (1991) MRC European Carotid Surgery Trial: interim results for symptomatic patients with severe (70–99%) or with mild (0–29%) carotid stenosis. *Lancet.* **337**: 1235–43.

4   North American Symptomatic Carotid Endarterectomy Trial Collaborators (1991) Beneficial effect of carotid endarterectomy in symptomatic patients with high-grade carotid stenosis. *NEJM.* **325**: 445–53.

5   Winslow CM, Solomon DH, Chassin MR, Kosecoff J, Merrick NJ and Brook RH (1988) The appropriateness of carotid endarterectomy. *NEJM.* **318**: 721–7.

6   World Health Organisation (1978) *Cerebrovascular Disease: a clinical and research classification.* Offset Series No. 43. World Health Organisation, Geneva.

7   Ebrahim S (1998) There are no short cuts to finding out what works – population laboratories are essential tools. *Trop Med Int Health.* **3**: 256–7.

8   Murray CJL and Lopez AD (2000) *Progress and Directions in Refining the Global Burden of Disease Approach.* WHO discussion document; http://www.who.int/whosis/guides/guidemebod.htm. Accessed February 2001.

9   Tilling K (2001) Capture-recapture methods in epidemiology. *Int J Epidemiol.* **30**: 12–14.

10 Dennis M, Wellwood I and Warlow C (1997) Are simple questions a valid measure of outcome after stroke? *Cerebrovasc Dis.* **7**: 22–7.

11 Stroke Unit Trialists' Collaboration (2000) Organised inpatient (stroke unit) care for stroke (Cochrane Review). In: *The Cochrane Library. Issue 4.* Update Software, Oxford.

12 Smeeth L and Ebrahim S (2000) DINS, PINS and things – clinical and population perspectives on treatment effects. *BMJ.* **321**: 952–3.

Useful definitions

These definitions are taken from Last JM (ed.) (1988) *Dictionary of Epidemiology* (2e). Oxford University Press, Oxford.

Age standardisation

A procedure for adjusting rates (e.g. death rates), designed to minimise the effects of differences in age composition when comparing rates for different populations.

Bias

Deviation of results or inferences from the truth, or processes leading to such deviation. Any trend in the collection, analysis, interpretation, publication or review of data that can lead to conclusions that are systematically different from the truth. The ways in which deviation from the truth can occur include the following:

1 systematic (one-sided) variation of measurements from the true values (*syn.*, systematic error)
2 variation of statistical summary measures (means, rates, measures of association, etc.) from their true values as a result of systematic variation of measurements, other flaws in data collection, or flaws in study design or analysis
3 deviation of inferences from the truth as a result of flaws in study design, data collection, or the analysis or interpretation of results
4 a tendency of procedures (in study design, data collection, analysis, interpretation, review or publication) to yield results or conclusions that depart from the truth
5 prejudice leading to the conscious or unconscious selection of study procedures that depart from the truth in a particular direction, or to one-sidedness in the interpretation of results.

The term 'bias' does not necessarily carry an imputation of prejudice or other subjective factors, such as the experimenter's desire for a particular outcome. This differs from conventional usage in which bias refers to a partisan point of view.

Many varieties of bias have been described.*

Bias, ascertainment

Systematic error arising from the kind of individuals or patients (e.g. slightly ill, moderately ill, acutely ill) that the individual observer is seeing. Also systematic error arising from the diagnostic process (which may be determined by the culture, customs or individual idiosyncrasy of the person providing care for the patient).

Bootstrap

A technique for estimating the variance and the bias of an estimator by repeatedly drawing random samples with replacement from the observations at hand. One applies the estimator to each sample drawn, thus obtaining a set of estimates. The observed variance of this set is the bootstrap estimate of variance. The difference between the average of the set of estimates and the original estimate is the bootstrap estimate of bias.

Case fatality rate

The proportion of cases of a specified condition which are fatal within a specified time.

Case fatality rate (usually expressed as a percentage) =

$$\frac{\text{Number of deaths from a disease (in a given period)}}{\text{Number of diagnosed cases of that disease (in the same period)}} \times 100.$$

This definition can lead to paradox when more individuals die of the disease than develop it during a given period. For instance, chemical poisoning that is slowly but inexorably fatal may cause many individuals to develop the disease over a relatively short period of time, but the deaths may not occur until some years later, and may be spread over a period of years during which there are no new cases. Thus when calculating the case fatality rate, it is necessary to acknowledge that the time dimension varies.

---

*Sackett DL (1979) Bias in analytic research. *J Chron Dis.* **32**: 51–63.

It may be brief (e.g. covering only the period of stay in a hospital), of finite duration (e.g. one year), or of longer duration still. The term 'case fatality rate' is then better replaced by a term such as 'survival rate'.

Comorbidity

Disease(s) that coexist(s) in a study participant in addition to the index condition that is the subject of study.

Confidence interval

A range of values for a variable of interest (e.g. a rate), constructed so that this range has a specified probability of including the true value of the variable. The specified probability is called the confidence level, and the end points of the confidence interval are called the confidence limits.

Confounding (from the latin *confundere*, to mix together)

1 A situation in which the effects of two processes are not separated. The distortion of the apparent effect of an exposure on risk brought about by the association with other factors that can influence the outcome.
2 A relationship between the effects of two or more causal factors as observed in a set of data, such that it is not logically possible to separate the contribution that any single causal factor has made to an effect.
3 A situation in which a measure of the effect of an exposure on risk is distorted because of the association of exposure with other factor(s) that influence the outcome under study.

Healthcare

Those services provided to individuals or communities by agents of the health services or professions, for the purpose of promoting, maintaining, monitoring or restoring health. Healthcare is broader than and not limited to medical care, which implies therapeutic action by or under the supervision of a physician. The term is sometimes extended to include self-care.

Health services research

The integration of epidemiological, sociological, economic and other analytical sciences in the study of health services. Health services research is usually concerned with relationships between *need*, *demand*, supply, use and *outcome* of health services. The aim of health services research is evaluation. The following components of evaluative health services research are distinguished:

- evaluation of *structure*, concerned with resources, facilities and manpower
- evaluation of *process*, concerned with matters such as where, by whom and how healthcare is provided
- evaluation of *output*, concerned with the amount and nature of health services provided
- evaluation of *outcome*, concerned with the results (i.e. whether individuals using health services experience measurable benefits such as improved survival or reduced disability).

Health status index

A set of measurements designed to detect short-term fluctuations in the health of members of a population. These measurements generally include physical function, emotional well-being, activities of daily living, feelings, etc. Most indexes require the use of carefully composed questions designed with reference to matters of fact rather than shades of opinion. The results are usually expressed by means of a numerical score that gives a profile of the well-being of the individual.

Incidence (*syn.*, incident number)

The number of instances of illness commencing, or of individuals falling ill, during a given period in a specified population.* More generally, the number of new events (e.g. new cases of a disease in a defined population) within a specified period of time. The term incidence is sometimes used to denote *incidence rate*.

---

* World Health Organisation (1966) Prevalence and incidence. *WHO Bull.* **35**: 783–4.

Incidence rate

The rate at which new events occur in a population. The numerator is the number of new events that occur in a defined period. The denominator is the population at risk of experiencing the event during this period, sometimes expressed as person-time. The incidence rate most often used in public health practice is calculated by the following formula:

$$\frac{\text{number of new events in a specified period}}{\text{number of individuals exposed to risk during this period}} \times 10^n.$$

In a dynamic population, the denominator is the average size of the population, often the estimated population at the mid-period. If the period is a year, this is the annual incidence rate. This rate is an estimate of the person-time incidence rate (i.e. the rate per 10^n person-years). If the rate is low, as with many chronic diseases, it is also a good estimate of the cumulative incidence rate. In follow-up studies with no censoring, the incidence rate is calculated by dividing the number of new cases in a specified period by the initial size of the cohort of individuals being followed. This is equivalent to the cumulative incidence rate during the period. If the number of new cases during a specified period is divided by the sum of the person-time units at risk for all individuals during the period, the result is the person-time incidence rate.

Minimum data (core) set (*syn.,* uniform basic data set)

A widely agreed upon and generally accepted set of terms and definitions constituting a core of data acquired for medical records and employed for developing statistics suitable for diverse types of analyses and users. Such sets have been developed for birth and death certificates, ambulatory care, hospital care and long-term care.

Morbidity

Any departure, subjective or objective, from a state of physiological or psychological well-being. In this sense, *sickness, illness* and morbid condition are similarly defined and synonymous.

The WHO Expert Committee on Health Statistics noted in its Sixth Report (published in 1959) that morbidity could be measured in terms of three units:

1 individuals who were ill
2 the illnesses (periods or spells of illness) that these individuals experienced
3 the duration (days, weeks, etc.) of these illnesses.

Prevalence

The number of instances of a given disease or other condition in a given population at a designated time, sometimes used to mean prevalence rate. When used without qualification, the term usually refers to the situation at a specified point in time (point prevalence).

Quality of care

A level of performance or accomplishment that characterises the healthcare provided. Ultimately, measures of the quality of care always depend upon value judgements, but there are ingredients and determinants of quality that can be measured objectively. These ingredients and determinants have been classified by Donabedian* into measures of structure (e.g. manpower, facilities), process (e.g. diagnostic and therapeutic procedures) and outcome (e.g. case fatality rates, disability rates, and levels of patient satisfaction with the service).

Questionnaire

A predetermined set of questions used to collect data (clinical data, social status, occupational group, etc.). This term is often applied to a self-completed survey instrument, as contrasted with an interview schedule.

Register, registry

In epidemiology, the term 'register' is applied to a file of data concerning all cases of a particular disease or other health-relevant condition in a defined population such that the cases can be related to a population base. With this information, incidence rates can be calculated. If the cases are regularly followed up, information on remission, exacerbation, prevalence and survival can also be obtained. The *register* is the actual document, and the *registry* is the system of ongoing registration.

---

*Donabedian A (1969) *A Guide to Medical Care Administration. Volume 2.* American Public Health Association, New York.

Standardised mortality (morbidity) ratio (SMR)

The ratio of the number of events observed in the study group or population to the number that would be expected if the study population had the same specific rates as the standard population, multiplied by 100.

Index